IMPORTANT

This book is intended not as a substitute for personal
medical advice but as a supplement to that advice for
the patient who wishes to understand more about his
or her condition.

Before taking any form of treatment
YOU SHOULD ALWAYS CONSULT YOUR MEDICAL
PRACTITIONER.

In particular (without limit) you should note that advances
in medical science occur rapidly and some information
about drugs and treatment contained in this booklet may
very soon be out of date.

Family Doctor Publications, PO Box 4664, Poole, Dorset BH15 1NN

ISBN-13: 978-1-903474-617
ISBN 10: 1-903474-612

20092011

Contents

Patient experiences

Sharing knowledge and experience of ill health

Many people who have experienced ill health are much wiser as a result.

On our website (www.familydoctor.co.uk) we are creating a resource where people who wish to know more about an illness or condition can learn from other people's experiences of that illness.

If you have had a health experience that may be useful to someone in a similar situation, we invite you to share this by clicking on the 'Patient Experience' tab at www.familydoctor.co.uk (see below).

- Your 'Patient Experience' will be completely anonymous – there will be no link back to you and we require no personal information from you.

- Your 'Patient Experience' will not be a forum or discussion – there is no opportunity for others to comment either positively or negatively on what you have written.

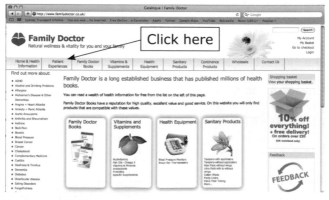

About the authors

Dr Nori Graham BM, Bch, FRCPsych, DUniv is Emeritus Consultant in the Psychiatry of Old Age at the Royal Free Hospital where she was responsible for many years for a community-oriented multidisciplinary service for older people with mental illness.

She was the National Chairman of the Alzheimer's Society for England from 1987 to 1994, and Chairman of Alzheimer's Disease International (ADI), the umbrella organisation of national Alzheimer associations worldwide, from 1996 to 2002. She is now Vice-President of the Alzheimer's Society, England and Honorary Vice-President of ADI.

In 1996 she was awarded an honorary doctorate for public services by the Open University.

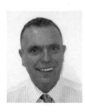

Dr James Warner BSc, MB BS, MD, MRCP, FRCPsych is a Consultant in Old Age Psychiatry at St Charles Hospital, London and Honorary Reader in Psychiatry at Imperial College London. He works in a team providing community assessment and treatment of older people with mental illness and dementia.

Dr Warner's academic interests include teaching and research into dementia. He is the author of over 50 scientific papers, several books and book chapters.

Dr Warner is a member of the old age psychiatry section committee of the World Psychiatric Association and trustee for the charity Dementia UK.

Introduction

Who is this book for?

- You think your memory is going?

- Your father/mother is behaving oddly?

- Is it Alzheimer's disease?

- Is Alzheimer's disease the same as dementia?

If these are the sorts of questions that you are asking yourself, this book is for you. Dementia is a disease of the brain. First we define dementia before going on to list the symptoms. This chapter helps you decide whether you, a member of your family or a friend may have dementia.

Next we discuss treatment and how to get help, and after that we give some tips on how to make the best of life if you or a loved one is found to have dementia. Then we consider how future developments may change the outlook for people with dementia, and describe some common questions and give some answers. Finally, we describe how the brain works.

Some of that chapter is a bit technical; you may decide to skip it.

There is a lot of myth and misinformation about dementia. This book is intended for anyone who has, or may be worried that they or their family and friends have, dementia.

It is also for people who live or work with someone with dementia. We hope that by reading this book you will have a better understanding of what causes the illness and how it is diagnosed and treated.

What is dementia?

'Dementia' is a term used to describe any condition where a variety of different brain functions such as memory, thinking, recognition, language, planning and personality deteriorate over time.

Dementia is not part of normal ageing. Everyone gets more forgetful as they get older; that does not mean that they have dementia. The most common type of dementia is Alzheimer's disease, but there are several other types.

Who gets dementia?

Dementia is common. It is estimated that there are almost three-quarters of a million people with dementia in the UK and this number is rising. As people get older the risk of dementia increases rapidly. It is estimated that one in six people aged over 80 years has some type of dementia.

Dementia can affect anyone. Prominent people such as Ronald Reagan, Harold Wilson, Margaret Thatcher, Iris Murdoch, Terry Pratchett and many other well-known names from all walks of life have developed dementia. It is a global problem, occurring in all ethnic groups and social classes. No one is immune.

It is important to recognise when someone may have dementia. A swift and accurate diagnosis is important while people can still plan their lives and have a say in their treatment. Getting a diagnosis is also helpful to explain why someone isn't getting on as well as they used to and ensures that they get the necessary help. It is also reassuring to be told if you don't have dementia.

Facts and figures about dementia

Dementia is common; about one in every 90 people in the UK has dementia. In 2008, it was estimated that there were 700,000 people in the UK with dementia and this will rise to 1 million by 2025.

Dementia is rare below the age of 65, but can occur in people as young as 30. About 1 in 20 people over the age of 65 has dementia, rising to about 1 in 6 of people aged over 80. Dementia is becoming more common because the biggest risk factor for dementia is getting older and people are living longer.

About two-thirds of people with dementia live at home. Almost three-quarters of people living in care homes have dementia. People who develop dementia often live for many years with the condition. It is not uncommon for someone to live seven to ten years after a diagnosis and then to die of something else. Nearly everyone who has dementia will get worse over time and many people will eventually need to be cared for because they cannot live safely alone.

Diagnosing and treating dementia

The prospect of receiving a diagnosis of dementia is frightening. Other conditions such as depression and some physical illnesses (for example, Parkinson's disease) can look like dementia. Dementia can be diagnosed only after careful assessment by a doctor.

In the last 15 years there has been a great deal of research into treatments of dementia and drugs are now available to treat memory loss and problems with thinking. There has also been a lot of progress in understanding how someone with dementia, and families and carers, can be supported.

In this book we describe how dementia is diagnosed and treated. It is important to remember that not all the services and facilities described in this book are available in all areas.

Living with dementia

People with dementia can have a good quality of life with help, support and quality care. Dementia is not just about memory loss. Many other problems can occur during the course of the illness including anxiety, depression, wandering, incontinence and aggression. These can be helped too, and we have included practical advice to help cope with the day-to-day problems that can occur in dementia.

Throughout this book we have used examples to illustrate some of the problems and difficulties. Although these are based on real patients, we have changed the details to ensure anonymity.

KEY POINTS

- The term 'dementia' is used to describe the symptoms that occur when the brain is affected by specific diseases and conditions

- Dementia is not part of normal ageing

- Dementia is common, affecting almost 700,000 people in the UK

What is dementia?

Case study – Mary

Mary, a retired factory worker, is 79 and lives alone after her husband died 3 years ago. Mary is becoming increasingly worried about her memory. Recently she went shopping and left her shopping trolley in the library when she popped in to return a book. On another occasion she forgot her PIN number when collecting her pension from the post office.

She visited her doctor because she thought she was developing Alzheimer's disease. Dr Thomas listened carefully to her problems and ordered some tests. It turned out Mary did not have dementia. 'As we get older our memory does get worse,' Dr Thomas told her. 'But a problem with memory alone does not mean someone is developing Alzheimer's disease, or any other dementia.'

This chapter explains what dementia is, and outlines the common types of dementia and conditions that can mimic it.

Defining dementia

Dementia is a term that is applied to several different conditions that affect the brain. Just like the word 'arthritis' refers to many different causes of joint pain, there are several different types of dementia, with subtly different symptoms. The most common cause of dementia is Alzheimer's disease, but there are many other causes.

Most kinds of dementia have similar symptoms including:

- Loss of memory

- Problems with thinking and planning

- Difficulties with language

- Failure to recognise people or objects

- A change of personality.

Our brains (if we think about what our brains do) have many different functions. Making a cup of tea might seem a simple task but in fact this is quite a complex task and provides examples of several different brain functions:

1. We imagine a cup of tea (abstract thinking) and decide to make one (motivation).

2. We may ask whoever is with us if they want a cup (language).

3. We plan making the tea ensuring that things are done in the right order, putting the tea in before the boiling water (executive function).

4. We remember where the tea, sugar and milk are stored (memory).

5. We put the kettle on and gather the ingredients (motor function).

6. We listen for the kettle (hearing), ensuring that we don't get distracted with some other task (attention and concentration).

7. We carefully pour (coordination) just the right amount of water (judgement) on to the tea.

8. We may then may add milk and sugar to the cup, in the right order (planning).

9. We wait until it has cooled sufficiently (judgement) and we enjoy the tea (taste).

10. All the way through we have probably spoken and acted in a similar manner to how we usually do (personality).

Most people reading this book have, at some time or another, made a mistake when making tea. For example, putting tea bags in the fridge and milk in the cupboard instead of the other way round, popping into the next room to ask someone if they want a cuppa and totally forgetting what you wanted to ask or making a cup of tea and forgetting to drink it.

This does not mean that you have dementia. When someone has dementia, usually several of the different brain functions outlined above begin to go wrong, and not just once but repeatedly over time.

So dementia could be defined as:

Persistent, progressive problems with more than one aspect of brain function (such as language, planning, motivation, memory or personality).

The *International Classification of Diseases* defines dementia as follows: each of the following, present for at least six months in someone who has no impairment of consciousness:

- Decline in memory

- Decline in other cognitive abilities such as judgement, thinking, planning

- Decline in emotional control (for example, irritability) or motivation.

Symptoms of dementia

In many types of dementia, problems with memory and complex thinking are the first symptoms. The memory loss is usually for recent things. So someone may have a clear recollection for things that happened years ago, but cannot remember things that happened a few hours or days ago.

Dementia must be differentiated from acute (sudden-onset) causes of confusion. Dementia comes on over months or years; if someone becomes confused over a matter of hours or days this is unlikely to be a dementia.

Acute confusion is usually the result of another physical cause such as:

- Infection (for example, chest or urine infection)

- A reaction to medicines

- Pain or constipation

- Stroke

- Other physical cause.

Having dementia is a risk factor for getting a more acute confusional state, but, in every case, if someone gets suddenly confused (or more confused), he or she should see a doctor to try to find the cause of the acute confusion.

People who have dementia can also become more confused if there is a change in routine, such as going on holiday or going into hospital.

Types of dementia

There are a large number of different types and causes of dementia but the great majority of people have one of four types:

1. Alzheimer's disease

2. Vascular dementia

3. Lewy body dementia

4. Frontotemporal dementia.

We shall concentrate on these four. Together, Alzheimer's disease and vascular dementia cause about 90 per cent of all cases of dementia.

Brain scans and special tests of brain function (cognitive tests) may help doctors tell what type of dementia a person has. However, the only sure way of telling what type of dementia is present is by doing a brain biopsy (removing a small piece of brain tissue and looking at it under a microscope). This is very rarely done.

Alzheimer's disease
Case study – Gordon
Gordon was 74 when his wife, Liz, first began to notice something was wrong. Looking back, Liz first noticed

that Gordon was not looking after his allotment properly. He had been a very keen gardener, often winning prizes for his vegetables. However, recently Gordon had made some mistakes: planting seeds at the wrong time, forgetting to water his plants and letting the weeds get out of control. Neighbours commented that his allotment was a mess.

At first Liz thought Gordon was just bored with gardening, but then other things happened. Gordon was driving back from the supermarket when he suddenly took a wrong turn and went the wrong way up a one-way street.

A few weeks later he got into a muddle with his bank statement and flew into a rage – a very rare thing for him to do.

Liz tried to get Gordon to see the doctor but he was adamant that there was nothing wrong. Eventually Liz called Dr Blunt herself, but he told her it was probably just old age and advised her not to worry.

Over the next year things got worse. Gordon began to dress less smartly, sometimes wearing the same clothes until Liz reminded him to change. He began to repeat conversations and would often ask Liz the same question several times over.

He gave up the allotment and would sit for hours doing very little. Liz insisted Gordon went to the doctor and this time she went with him and the doctor took a careful history of Gordon's problems and referred Gordon to the local memory assessment service.

After visiting Gordon and Liz at home and doing some tests, the consultant diagnosed Gordon as having Alzheimer's disease.

Alzheimer's disease is the most common form of dementia; about two-thirds of people with dementia have Alzheimer's disease. This disease was first described over 100 years ago by Alois Alzheimer who reported on a condition in a woman in her 50s. His description shows the range of symptoms that may develop in this condition:

> One of the first disease symptoms of a 51-year-old woman was a strong feeling of jealousy towards her husband. Very soon she showed rapidly increasing memory impairments; she could not find her way about her home, she dragged objects to and fro, hid herself, or sometimes thought that people were out to kill her; then she would start to scream loudly. From time to time she was completely delirious, dragging her blankets and sheets to and fro, calling for her husband and daughter, and seeming to have auditory hallucinations. Often she would scream for hours and hours in a horrible voice.

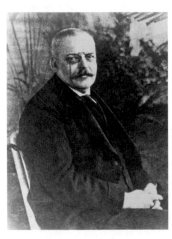

Portrait of Alois Alzheimer 1864

Alzheimer's disease usually begins with very mild symptoms. The first symptoms are often mild memory loss, which can be difficult to tell from normal forgetfulness as a result of getting older.

Mild confusion (for example, with managing bills) and problems with use of language may also be present early in the illness. Alzheimer's disease usually starts slowly and with very mild symptoms; it is rare to find someone where the onset can be dated to a particular time, and someone may have the condition for a year or two before it is diagnosed.

Alzheimer's disease also tends to progress slowly. As the disease gets worse, people may have a range of different symptoms (see page 33) and may eventually become very disabled, needing round-the-clock help.

What happens to the brain in Alzheimer's disease?
Scientists now know quite a lot about what happens to the brains of people with Alzheimer's disease. The brain is made up of millions of nerve cells (among other things), which enable us to think and remember.

In a brain affected by Alzheimer's disease an abnormal protein called amyloid is made (for reasons that are not fully understood). Microscopic amounts of this amyloid protein are laid down in the outer layers of the brain in clumps called plaques.

These plaques are thought to affect the health of nerve cells or neurons. Neurons contain a protein called tau, which is involved in maintaining the shape of the nerve cell. Affected neurons begin to make an abnormal form of tau. This abnormal form of tau is thought to result in a change in structure of the cells.

Some nerve cells die and collapse in on themselves, creating clumps called tangles. These tangles, and

Brain tissue under the microscope

Brain tissue affected by Alzheimer's disease showing tangles and plaques.

Amyloid plaque

Neurofibrillary tangles

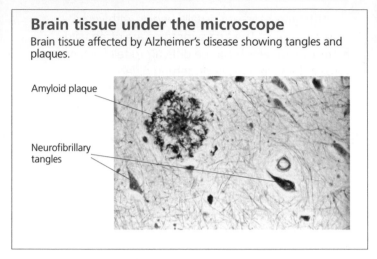

the plaques of amyloid protein, are visible under the microscope and are the hallmarks of Alzheimer's disease.

Certain parts of the brain, especially the temporal lobe (a part of the brain where memory is stored) shrink as a result of the death of neurons. This shrinkage can be seen on some brain scans, and this can help doctors make a diagnosis.

The nerve cells in the brain communicate with each other using chemicals called transmitters. In Alzheimer's disease, there is less of some of these transmitters, and some treatments for Alzheimer's disease are aimed at increasing the levels of these chemicals (see 'Treatments for dementia', page 50).

What causes Alzheimer's disease?

Little is known about what triggers the process that leads people to develop Alzheimer's disease. Alzheimer's disease may run in families, but this is

The process of Alzheimer's disease

1. Normal brain

Neurons within the brain transmit electrical messages to other parts of the body using chemicals called transmitters.

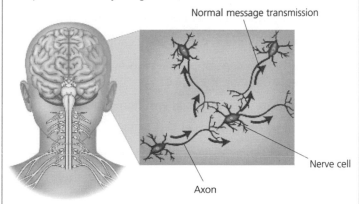

Normal message transmission

Nerve cell

Axon

2. Brain with Alzheimer's disease

In Alzheimer's disease areas of the brain tissue are damaged and this interferes with message transmission, causing the symptoms of the disease.

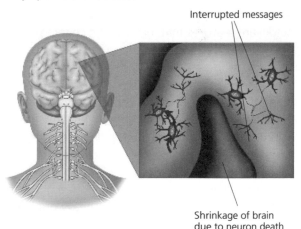

Interrupted messages

Shrinkage of brain due to neuron death

Key features of Alzheimer's disease

- The most common cause of dementia
- Slightly more common in women than in men
- Affects 26 million people worldwide
- Over 90 per cent of people with Alzheimer's disease are over the age of 70
- Slow start with very mild symptoms initially
- Memory often affected first
- Smooth progression, often over many years
- People often live 10 years or even more after diagnosis

nearly always only in those very rare cases when the disease begins in younger people

Risk factors for developing Alzheimer's disease
Risk factors are features that increase the chances that a person will develop dementia. The single most important risk for developing Alzheimer's disease is increasing age; as we age beyond 70 the risk for developing the disease increases considerably.

Other risk factors, such as being female, repeated head injury (such as in boxers), high blood pressure, being overweight and not exercising, increase the chances only a little.

Drinking small amounts of alcohol (about a glass of wine) regularly may reduce the risk, but heavy drinking may increase it.

Factors that may increase the risk for Alzheimer's disease

- Older age
- Being female
- Genetics (hereditary factors)
- Head injury
- Less education
- High blood pressure
- High cholesterol
- Diabetes
- Obesity

A family history of Alzheimer's disease

A very small number of people develop Alzheimer's disease in middle age. In these 'young-onset' cases the disease may be caused by an abnormal gene that is passed from one generation to the next. Genes, which are made up of DNA, are stored in chromosomes, which are found in every cell in the body.

Genes transmit information (for example, characteristics such as skin and eye colour) from one generation to the next. Each person has a pair of genes for each characteristic. Some genes develop abnormalities, called mutations, and these abnormal genes can transmit diseases.

Gene mutations on different chromosomes (chromosomes 1, 14 and 21) have been found that can transmit Alzheimer's disease in this way. If a person has one of these gene mutations they will, on average, pass it to half their children.

Anyone who inherits one of these genes is highly likely to develop Alzheimer's disease, often in their 40s or 50s. However, this is incredibly rare; Alzheimer's disease due to these abnormal genes accounts for less than 1 in every 1,000 cases.

If there is a strong family history of Alzheimer's disease starting before the age 60, then doctors may be able to test whether healthy family members are carrying the Alzheimer's disease gene.

The vast majority of people with Alzheimer's disease do not have the type that is passed on from generation to generation by a single gene.

In this 'non-inherited' form of the disease, the risk to close relatives is still higher than for a person of a similar age who has no family history of Alzheimer's disease. For example, someone with no family history has about a 1 in 50 chance of developing Alzheimer's disease during his or her seventieth year. This risk would increase to about 1 in 20 in someone with a close relative who did have Alzheimer's disease. The risk is higher still when two close family members are affected.

Vascular dementia
Case study – Frank

My name is Frank. I am 69 and worked for many years as a taxi driver. I first noticed something was wrong when I began to take punters on the wrong route while at work. I was always proud of my 'knowledge' of the streets, so this worried me.

Then one day I felt a bit dizzy and had problems finding the right words to speak. It only lasted 20 minutes or so but I was bothered so went to my GP. By this time my memory was quite bad. My GP organised for me to see a specialist very quickly.

After he did some tests the specialist told me my brain scan showed that I have a poor blood supply to the brain and as a result I have had a lot of mini-strokes ('infarcts' he called them). I didn't realise!

He also tested my memory and said I am in the early stages of vascular dementia. I also have high cholesterol and high blood pressure. I am on aspirin and tablets to control my blood pressure. I don't feel too bad but I have had to give up work and get under the missus' feet a bit.

The second most common cause of dementia is vascular dementia. Around one in four people with dementia has this condition, either on its own or combined with Alzheimer's disease (sometimes called mixed dementia).

Vascular dementia (sometimes known as multi-infarct dementia or vascular cognitive impairment) refers to dementia that occurs because the blood supply to the brain is not as good as it should be or the blood supply to a region of the brain has been interrupted.

The brain needs a great deal of blood to carry oxygen to the nerve cells and receives around a fifth of the blood that is pumped around the body.

Blood is pumped from the heart through arteries. As these arteries travel deeper into the brain they divide into a multitude of smaller vessels called arterioles. Each arteriole feeds a small section of the brain.

Normally the walls of these arteries and arterioles are smooth, but they may become thickened by fatty deposits called atheroma.

When this happens, the artery narrows and the wall becomes roughened. Less blood can get through the narrowed artery, and sometimes the artery wall may

The process of atheroma

Atheroma is the process by which fat is deposited on the inside walls of blood vessels. The deposits can grow to such an extent that they restrict blood flow.

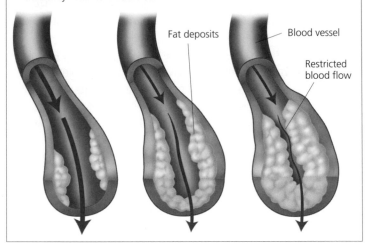

Fat deposits

Blood vessel

Restricted blood flow

develop a clot of blood and block off completely. If this happens in the brain it results in a stroke or infarct.

Sometimes a short-lived interruption to the blood supply to a region of the brain may not cause any lasting effect. This is known as a transient ischaemic attack (TIA). A stroke causes lasting damage.

If the blockage resulting in a stroke is in a small artery or arteriole, the resulting stroke may be very small with minor symptoms, but a blockage in a large artery can cause death of a large region of brain and result in death or major symptoms including paralysis, loss of speech or blindness.

Vascular dementia may arise either because the blood supply to the brain is reduced as a result of narrowing of the arteries caused by atheroma, or because of a stroke or series of strokes. Often people

Stroke

The most common cause of a stroke is a thrombosis – when a blood vessel supplying vital nutrients to the brain becomes blocked with a blood clot.

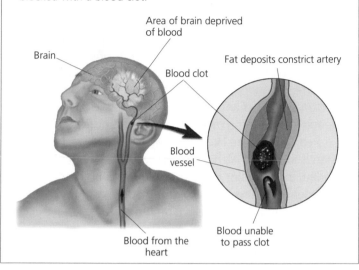

Area of brain deprived of blood

Brain

Blood clot

Fat deposits constrict artery

Blood vessel

Blood unable to pass clot

Blood from the heart

have a history of TIAs or several small strokes before they develop vascular dementia.

Vascular dementia may begin more abruptly than Alzheimer's disease and may get worse in phases (called step-wise progression) rather than gradually. People with this type of dementia, especially in the early stages,

Key features of vascular dementia

- Second most common cause of dementia
- Slightly more common in men than in women
- Caused by a poor blood supply to the brain
- Often has a sudden start and gets worse in steps

may have intervals (which may be long or short) when they are much more 'with it'.

Symptoms of vascular dementia
The symptoms of vascular dementia can vary depending on which parts of the brain are affected by the poor blood supply. A brain scan can show what areas of the brain are affected.

Often memory and language are affected early, and personality can change early in the disease (for example, people can become more irritable or unmotivated).

People are more likely to be aware of their dementia than if they have Alzheimer's disease. The main finding in the brains of people with vascular dementia is evidence of a reduced flow of blood – often with numerous tiny strokes visible on brain scans.

Risk factors for vascular dementia

- People who smoke
- People with diabetes
- High blood pressure
- Obesity

Lewy body dementia
Case study – Roy
Roy is 75 and lives alone. He began to have difficulties about three years ago. His first symptom was seeing things that a few seconds later he realised were not there. He often said he saw cats sitting on a chair in his living room but when he looked again they had gone.

About six months before this, Roy developed a shake on his left hand and had problems walking. His doctor had diagnosed early Parkinson's disease.

When Roy's daughter visited him for a week she got quite worried. She found that Roy was getting up at night and staring at the front door. When she tried to talk to him he seemed unaware that she was there and could not remember anything the following day. She also noticed that Roy seemed quite confused at times, but virtually normal just a few hours later. At his daughter's prompting Roy went to the doctor who diagnosed Lewy body dementia.

Lewy body dementia accounts for about 1 in 20 cases of dementia. It is quite different from Alzheimer's disease and vascular dementia. Early on, people with Lewy body dementia usually have symptoms of Parkinson's disease (shaking, especially in the hands, stiffness and reduced mobility). They also experience hallucinations, often seeing things that are not there (such as people or animals).

Key features of Lewy body dementia

- Third most common cause of dementia in the UK

- More common in men

- People have fluctuating confusion – often with spells where they may seem almost normal (at least early on)

- Features include symptoms of Parkinson's disease and visual hallucinations

- Risk of falls and poor mobility

Lewy bodies

Microscopic examination of the brain of a patient with Lewy body dementia shows a loss of cells and the presence of protein structures called Lewy bodies in some of the surviving nerve cells.

Microscope section of a nerve cell

Nerve cell

Cerebrum   Cerebellum

Brain stem

Spinal cord

Lewy body

Electron micrograph of a Lewy body

The difficulties in thinking and memory are similar to Alzheimer's disease but may vary from hour to hour. People with Lewy body dementia are prone to falls and may have restless nights when they move a lot while apparently dreaming.

People who have had Parkinson's disease for many years seem to have a higher risk of developing dementia that is similar to Lewy body dementia.

In common with other types of dementia, older age is a risk factor for developing Lewy body dementia. Other risk factors include being male and having a family history of the disease.

Very little is known about what causes Lewy body dementia. If scientists look at the brains of people with Lewy body dementia they find microscopic lumps of protein in the nerve cells in the brain, called Lewy bodies. These protein deposits disrupt the normal functioning of nerve cells.

Frontotemporal dementia
Case study – Adam

Adam is 56, divorced and living alone. He was a successful executive in an advertising firm. About four years ago colleagues noticed that Adam was making increasingly outlandish and daring decisions at work.

Some customers liked his 'off-the-wall' suggestions so colleagues didn't worry too much. However, Adam, who had always prided himself on his punctuality, began to miss meetings and turn up late for work. He began to swear and make rude comments to people, both quite uncharacteristic things for him to do.

When Adam began making inappropriate sexual comments to female colleagues, some friends dismissed his behaviour as caused by the 'male menopause'. One of his friends got really worried and went to see Adam at home and found that he was living in a mess, with stacks of rubbish and boxes of things that Adam had bought on impulse but never unpacked.

Adam appeared quite unbothered about all this and seemed quite bewildered when the friend expressed concern. Finally, his friends persuaded him to see a doctor. Investigations showed that Adam had a type of dementia called frontotemporal dementia.

About 1 in 50 people with dementia has the fronto-temporal type. People with frontotemporal dementia tend to be younger than those with other types of dementia. Of all the types of dementia, frontotemporal dementia is often the most difficult to spot, usually because it affects people in their 50s when dementia is rarely suspected.

The main area of the brain affected is the frontal lobe, resulting in changes in personality, motivation and increasingly odd or uninhibited behaviour. People affected by this type of dementia may have problems concentrating, develop obsessional 'rituals' and become aggressive. Sometimes people have problems finding the right words, or their speech becomes repetitive or less meaningful.

The areas of the brain mainly involved in memory are affected fairly late in the disease so memory may appear normal at first. The symptoms of frontotemporal dementia are subtle at first and can develop over a very long period of time. Symptoms may be put down to 'midlife crisis' or 'menopause'.

Frontotemporal dementia is usually diagnosed after a brain scan, which may show considerable thinning (atrophy) of the frontal lobe, whereas other parts of the brain may look normal. Cognitive tests can show specific difficulties with tasks dependent on the frontal lobe such as concentration or responding to changing patterns of information.

Some frontotemporal dementia is genetically inherited – about half of all people with it have a family history. It is not known what causes the non-genetic form of the disease.

Dementia related to alcohol

Drinking small amounts of alcohol, say one unit (pub measure) a day, is thought to reduce the risk of developing dementia. However, heavy drinking (several units a day) can increase the chance of dementia.

One specific condition related to prolonged heavy drinking is known as Korsakoff's syndrome. Korsakoff's syndrome usually has a sudden onset, often occurring after a period of acute confusion. Individuals are unable to lay down any new memories following the onset of this condition, although memories for events before the disease are often unaffected.

The result is a very disabling amnesia, but without the other symptoms of dementia (for example, language and thinking difficulties or personality change) described in this book. Korsakoff's syndrome is thought to result from a deficiency of a vitamin called thiamine. There is damage to a very specific part of the brain (called the mamillary bodies) although the rest of the brain may seem unaffected on a scan.

In addition to Korsakoff's syndrome, prolonged heavy use of alcohol probably also causes a dementia with symptoms similar to Alzheimer's disease. Some authorities have estimated that up to 10% of all cases of dementia are related to alcohol.

Rarer types of dementia

There are a very large number of rarer causes of dementia, some of which are described below.

Parkinson's disease dementia

This is similar to Lewy body dementia but the dementia comes on many years after the person develops Parkinson's disease. Eventually about one in four people with Parkinson's disease will develop dementia. People tend to have fewer problems with memory, and more apathy and difficulty with planning compared with someone with Alzheimer's disease (see Family Doctor Book *Understanding Parkinson's Disease*).

Huntington's disease

This is an inherited disorder that usually begins between age 30 and 50. People with this condition usually develop severe problems with movement and have difficulty controlling their limbs. Anxiety and depression are common. Dementia usually presents with frontal symptoms (problems with planning and thinking and changes in personality) rather than memory problems.

Creutzfeldt–Jakob disease

There are several subtypes of this very rare disease, which affects about 50 people in the UK each year. Typical Creutzfeldt–Jakob disease (CJD) generally occurs in people who are elderly.

It is caused by a protein called a prion, although the disease can develop many decades after infection. The risk factors for this condition are not fully known, but a small proportion of cases seem to run in families. There is rapid development of dementia, often with blindness and severe difficulties with movement. Death usually occurs within a year of developing the condition.

Variant CJD (vCJD) is rarer than CJD and usually occurs in much younger people, typically in their 20s and 30s. This variant may be related to bovine spongiform encephalopathy (BSE or mad cow disease). The vast majority of cases worldwide have occurred in the UK. People develop depression or anxiety, and problems with sensation and pain before they show signs of dementia.

HIV-related dementia
About 10 per cent of people with AIDS will eventually develop dementia, often late in the illness. The main features are slowing of mental processes and worsening memory. With antiretroviral treatments this is now rare.

Progressive supranuclear palsy
In this condition, the nerves controlling balance and movement are damaged, leading to loss of coordination, slurred speech and falls. There may also be personality change. Dementia often occurs after these other symptoms have developed.

Conditions that look like dementia
Case study – Anne
Anne is 74. Her husband died last year and since then Anne has been getting more and more forgetful. She had to stop playing cards in the local bridge club because she could not concentrate on the game. Then she forgot that she was due to organise the teas at a local Women's Institute meeting – a very embarrassing mistake.

Since then things have gone from bad to worse. She has lost her energy and found even simple things, like hanging out the washing, difficult to do. Eventually she spent more and more time just sitting at home doing nothing. She could not remember the plot of the book she was reading and lost interest in the TV.

When her doctor suggested that Anne may be depressed she didn't agree; she didn't feel sad or tearful.

She was worried that she had Alzheimer's disease, having seen a friend develop it a couple of years earlier.

However, after a course of treatment for depression her energy levels and concentration returned and her memory began to improve. Three months on she is back playing bridge and doing the teas at the WI.

There are many conditions that cause slowly progressive memory loss and confusion that look like dementia. Some of these are treatable. This is one reason why it is so important for people who have symptoms such as memory loss or change in personality to see a doctor for a full check-up.

Conditions that can mimic dementia

- Depression
- Underactive thyroid gland (a gland in the neck that regulates metabolism)
- Parkinson's disease
- Acute confusional state (delirium)
- Some vitamin deficiencies (for example, vitamin B_{12})
- Some infections (for example, syphilis)
- Rarely, a brain tumour can look like dementia

Depression

Depression will affect one in three people at some point in their lives. In particular in older people it can be mistaken for dementia because many of the symptoms are the same.

People with depression may complain of feeling low or depressed, may lack energy or lose a sense of enjoyment. Often nothing can brighten them up.

Other symptoms include poor sleep (especially waking early), loss of appetite, poor concentration and memory. These are also common symptoms of dementia. An added complication is that people with dementia are even more likely to get depression as well – as many as half the people with dementia will get depressed.

Things that may point to depression rather than dementia include:

- Feeling worse in the morning (as a rule people with dementia tend to be brighter in the mornings)

- Having thoughts of guilt, worthlessness or suicide

- Low mood, which is sustained over weeks.

Underactive thyroid gland
Also called hypothyroidism, this can start gradually and be difficult to spot. People with this condition may feel cold all the time, their skin may get coarse and dry, and they generally feel tired and 'slowed up'. A blood test will confirm the diagnosis.

Parkinson's disease
This is quite a common disorder in older people. People with Parkinson's disease may notice shaking or tremor (which often starts in one hand), which is more noticeable when relaxing, and stiffness in their arms and legs. People with Parkinson's disease show less facial expression and may have problems walking.

Delirium/acute confusional state

Sometimes people can get confused over a matter of hours or days. This is not dementia but something that doctors call delirium, or acute confusional state.

One of the main differences is that delirium starts very quickly. Also, people with delirium may be drowsy or sleepy.

People who have delirium often change rapidly; for example, they may appear quite calm one minute and become very distressed, agitated or aggressive the next. They often hallucinate (see things that are not there). Behaviour is usually more disturbed at night.

Many things can cause delirium, commonly chest or urine infections, diabetes, prescribed medicines, alcohol or a stroke. If someone develops an acute confusion he or she should see a doctor or be taken to the hospital urgently.

KEY POINTS

- Dementia is a disease; it is not caused by normal ageing

- The most common type of dementia is Alzheimer's disease, although there are many other causes

- Many conditions look like dementia; anyone who develops symptoms of confusion should see a doctor

Symptoms of dementia

How dementia starts

Dementia often begins subtly; when people with dementia and their families look back on when the first symptoms started, it is often difficult to date.

Sometimes people first notice a problem when the person with dementia has his or her routine changed; for example, when they go on holiday or become ill. The death of a partner can sometimes reveal dementia in the surviving partner. Bereavement does not cause dementia but may reveal it because the person who has died had been helping out.

In the UK it is thought that only one in three people with dementia ever sees a doctor and gets a proper diagnosis. Of those who do, it often takes one to two years between the start of symptoms and someone seeing a doctor.

This is too long, and our advice is that, if you suspect that you, or someone close to you, is developing dementia, seek medical advice sooner rather than later. An accurate diagnosis of dementia rules out the possibility of a different treatable condition such as depression that may look like dementia.

It also allows people with dementia and carers to better plan and prepare for the future, for example by setting up a lasting power of attorney. It also allows earlier access to treatment and management advice.

The progression of dementia

Dementia is usually a progressive disease. It affects people in different ways. This is because the symptoms and the way in which they develop reflect personality, lifestyle, quality of relationships, and mental and physical health.

Symptoms vary with the different types of dementia but there are some broad similarities between them all. Most common are loss of memory and loss of practical abilities leading to a loss of independence and affecting social relationships.

The course of the disease is very variable. People may live with disease for over 20 years but it could be much less than this. In the end people with dementia usually die of some other condition such as a heart attack or an infection, which may be quite unconnected with the dementia.

Over recent years, better care and understanding have generally led to a greater expectation of life, and quality of life, for people with dementia.

Although dementia progresses at different rates in different people it is helpful to describe the progress of the disease at an early stage, as the disease progresses and at the late stage. This is a rough guide only. No one will have all the symptoms listed but this list can help people with dementia and their carers to understand what they are likely to expect and help them to plan for the future.

Early stage
Case study – Richard

When Richard and Bev looked back, there were several clues over the years. His love of gardening faded; sometimes he just seemed a bit vague; he stopped doing the crossword puzzle. The very first thing that they noticed was that Richard was less able to hold conversations on the phone. He was OK if he was making the call, but got quite confused if someone else was ringing him.

The onset of dementia is usually very gradual so that it is difficult to know when it actually starts. This stage is often overlooked and it is only when people are helped to look back in time that they realise that odd symptoms did occur but their significance had not been recognised or they had been excused as being part of normal ageing.

'It was such a shock. Looking back, he had been acting rather strangely, but nothing had led me to believe that he had Alzheimer's.'

A person in the early stage may:

- Become forgetful, especially of things that have just happened

- Lose their sense of time leading to missing appointments or not paying bills

- Show loss of interest and poor concentration

- Lose motivation:

  'He used to be so proud of his garden. Then over a year or so it just became a wilderness.'

- Become more withdrawn

- Have language problems with difficulty finding the right words

- Show odd behaviour:

  'The golf course was where some of the first signs of the disease showed up. He started to break the rules of the game. Friends started to avoid playing with him.'

- Have difficulty making decisions

- Be less engaged with family/company:

  'He just changed, just stopped being himself. He was less chatty and less happy. At first I thought he was depressed.'

- Be 'different' from their old self

- Show mood changes and be depressed or easily irritable:

  'Before diagnosis I had been puzzled by the problems of forgetfulness, lethargy and depression. At first I did not confide in my wife as I seemed to think it was all my fault and that I should accept the circumstances.'

Middle stage

This is a time when it is clear that a person has dementia and that it is affecting everyday functioning and ability to live independently. This can give rise to changes in behaviour often through frustration and a lack of understanding on the part of the person with the dementia and the carer.

The person with dementia at this stage may:

- Become more forgetful – might forget names of family and close friends and recent events, which can often give rise to repetitive questioning

- Wander out of the house and get lost

- Not be able to work out the difference between day and night and have difficulty sleeping

- Have difficulties understanding what is being said

- Have increased difficulty with speech

- Have problems with household tasks such as cleaning and cooking

- Need help with dressing, washing and reminding about going to the toilet

- Lose things and blame others for taking them

- Become aggressive

- Experience hallucinations.

Late stage

This is when the person with dementia has very serious memory problems and becomes completely dependent on others for their physical care. They may:

- Have great difficulty communicating

- Have poor or no recognition of family and friends

- Not understand what is said to them or what is going on around them

- Need help with eating

- Be incontinent of urine and faeces

- Have difficulty walking

- Have difficulty swallowing

- Be chair and bed bound.

This stage can last months or years depending on the physical health of the person and the quality of the care that the person is receiving. Death may be caused by infections, strokes or heart attacks.

Final stages

By this stage the person will be unable to speak or move properly; he or she will need full care including help with eating and drinking.

Often in the last stages swallowing becomes difficult. Even at this late stage the person may have some awareness of his or her surroundings and people around. It is not known how much people can understand in this situation. Almost certainly he or she will be able to feel pain (for example, from toothache or constipation) and will feel uncomfortable if hungry or dehydrated.

In the past some doctors have treated people with dementia differently because they have dementia. This is not appropriate; people with dementia should have the same rights to treatment and specialist care as any other citizen.

It is important to come to terms with dying from dementia and make plans for death. If you have dementia it is helpful to discuss what treatments you would, or would not, want to have when you reach the final stages.

It is often a very good idea to write your thoughts and wishes down, for example using an advance decision. It is also helpful to appoint a welfare attorney who will be able to make decisions for you when you are no longer able to. Details on how to do these can be found at the Office of the Public Guardian (see page 133).

The decisions that you may wish to make include whether you would want to die at home or in hospital and whether you would want resuscitation if your heart stops.

When writing an advance decision doctors have to follow your wishes if you decline a treatment, but you cannot force them to treat you if this goes against their professional judgement. For example, you can say you don't want antibiotics if you get a chest infection, but you cannot ask doctors to help hasten your death by giving morphine.

Diagnosis of dementia

Recognising the symptoms of dementia is the first step towards receiving a diagnosis and getting help. If you or your relative is worried that you are depressed or forgetful or showing any of the signs described above then going to your GP is the first thing to do.

Early and accurate diagnosis is helpful for several reasons:

- It provides an explanation for symptoms and odd behaviour and helps the people with dementia and their carers to be better equipped to deal with the disease and know what to expect as time goes on:

  'Its good to know what I have, although I cannot always understand it. The best thing is to feel loved and have friends. Please do not leave me alone.'

'The diagnosis cleared a lot of my fears and anxieties when I did not know what was happening. It helped me to give better care to my Mum.'

- It allows people to understand what is happening to them and to have some control over their life. For example, they can decide on treatments, write wills, take a holiday, see distant relatives, and set up financial and welfare powers of attorney.

- Appropriate support services and financial help can be put in place and help people to plan for the future:

'A diagnosis helped both of us put plans in place for her care. It also prepared me to be a better advocate for her when she was no longer able.'

- It can ensure that other problems that can lead to memory loss such as depression are dealt with appropriately

- For a number of people with dementia, and it is not possible yet to predict which ones, medication offers the possibility of slowing the disease process. Obviously if the diagnosis is not made for whatever reason, it is not possible to offer such treatment.

How the diagnosis is made

There is no simple test to make the diagnosis of dementia. A diagnosis is made by taking a careful account from the person with the problem and, even more importantly, from a close relative or friend.

Seeing the doctor

The first step to getting a diagnosis is to see a doctor;

this often takes some courage. Often the people with dementia do not see themselves as having any problems, so it may be necessary for someone to accompany them to the doctor.

If someone needs to see a doctor but refuses, then consider speaking directly with the general practitioner on his or her behalf. Often the GP will ask some questions about memory and difficulties with day-to-day tasks. They may organise some tests themselves but it may speed things up if they refer on to a local specialist.

Specialist referral
This will usually be to an:

- Old age psychiatrist (a doctor specialising in the mental disorders of old age)

- A neurologist (a specialist in diseases of the nervous system)

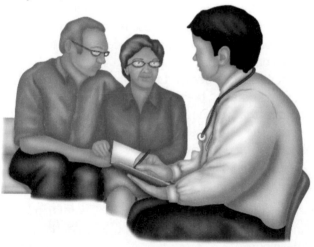

An early and accurate diagnosis of dementia can be helpful. The first step to getting a diagnosis is to see a doctor.

- A geriatrician (a specialist in medical diseases of older people).

Exactly which specialist someone is referred to will depend on their age, what symptoms they have and what services are available locally. Sometimes it may be necessary for a person to see more than one specialist; for example, a neurologist may ask an old age psychiatrist for a second opinion if symptoms of depression are present.

The specialist may see the person in a 'memory clinic' or hospital outpatients or go to see the person at home. Old age psychiatrists, in particular, often see a patient at home in the first instance. Seeing someone at home is not only usually more convenient for the patient but also allows the doctor to assess the home environment and gauge how well someone is coping at home.

Although the doctor will almost certainly want to ask someone else (usually a close relative or friend) for their account, they may want to speak to the person alone to begin with.

When seeing a doctor it is helpful to go prepared with some notes of the concerns that you have, the symptoms that you have noticed and when they started to occur. The assessment may take place on a single day, or may be done over a few weeks.

The doctor will normally ask questions about the following:

- The symptoms, especially when they were first noticed and how they have progressed and developed

- How they affect life and day-to-day tasks

- The person's past history including medical history and medication

- Description of the person's previous personality

- Family history

- The patient's views about the symptoms.

The doctor should build up an account of the person, known as a life story, so that he or she can see the difficulties in the context of the individual.

The assessment should include a physical examination to check that the heart and lungs are working properly, to check for signs of neurological illness such as Parkinson's disease or stroke, and to assess the risk of falls.

A psychological assessment should check for symptoms of depression, anxiety and psychosis (for example, having hallucinations).

Memory (cognitive) tests

It is common practice to carry out a simple memory test. One of the most commonly used is the Mini-Mental State Examination (MMSE), but several others are also used. Most tests take about 10 minutes. The doctor asks a series of questions including the date and where the person is now, and a test of comprehension, concentration and memory. He or she may also ask the person to repeat a phrase, copy a diagram and write a sentence.

The doctor may also do other tests such as naming animals or guessing heights of things. In many cases the doctor may refer for a more in-depth test of memory and thinking (called neuropsychometry), which is usually done by a psychologist (a specialist in mental processes such as memory). These tests can take up to an hour and give a detailed profile of changes in brain function and help map which parts of the brain (for example, the frontal lobe) are most affected in an individual. This can also estimate whether there has been a decrease compared with what would be expected for that individual.

Occupational therapist

Another person involved in the assessment may be an occupational therapist, who may conduct an assessment at home or in a special area in the hospital. This can be helpful in assessing skills with activities of daily living and areas where a person may need help or adaptations. It can also assess the environment and identify what changes or equipment may help maintain independence and reduce risks.

The assessment should check whether there are risks (for example, tripping on stairs or getting lost) and whether the person is getting enough food and can prepare meals. Looking in the fridge of someone who has dementia can reveal a great deal!

Social worker

A social worker may be involved in the assessment. Social workers can assess what practical help a person needs and arrange for this to be supplied or provide advice and information to help meet those needs. People with dementia are at risk of financial exploitation; finances may need safeguarding, through either appointeeship or the Court of Protection – something else that a social worker can help with.

Other investigations

Many people suspected of having dementia will have other investigations that are usually arranged by the specialist. These may include:

- A brain scan by CT (computed tomography)

- MRI (magnetic resonance imaging)

- PET (positron emission tomography).

These scans provide detailed images of the brain and can show areas of shrinkage or damage such as

Magnetic resonance imaging (MRI)

Magnetic resonance imaging (MRI) uses powerful magnets to align the atoms in the part of the body being studied. Radiowave pulses break the alignment, causing signals to be emitted from the atoms. These signals can be measured and a detailed image built up of the tissues and organs.

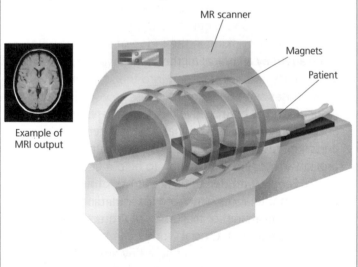

Example of MRI output

MR scanner

Magnets

Patient

Computed tomography (CT)

Computed tomography (CT) fires X-rays through the brain at different angles. The X-rays are picked up by receivers and the information analysed by a computer to create a picture of the brain.

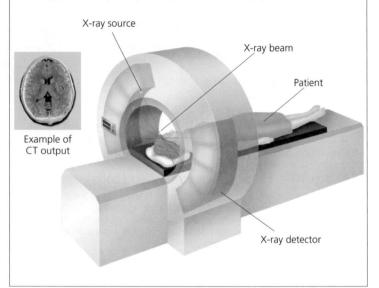

X-ray source

X-ray beam

Patient

Example of CT output

X-ray detector

that caused by a stroke. All the scans involve lying on a small trolley and being moved into the scanner.

MRI uses a strong magnetic pulse to visualise the structure of the brain and can produce very detailed images. An MR scan can take about half an hour; it is important to lie still and it can feel quite claustrophobic and noisy.

A CT scan uses a small dose of X-rays to create pictures of the brain. Although not as detailed as an MR scan, the image can still be useful. It takes only a few minutes to do a CT scan.

A PET scan involves injecting a tiny amount of radioactive substance into a vein and using this to

Positron emission tomography (PET)

A radionuclide is introduced into the body which is taken up by the nerve cells of the brain. The PET scan detects the emissions and using a computer builds up a picture of the brain's functioning.

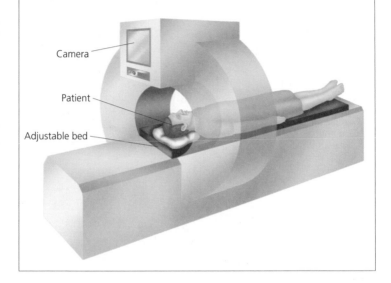

Camera

Patient

Adjustable bed

create an image of how the brain is working. PET scans are less common than MR and CT scans but may be used where the diagnosis is not clear.

The results of these scans can take some weeks to get back. Almost certainly the doctor will order some blood tests to check for anaemia, inflammation, vitamin levels, the health of the thyroid gland, and kidney and liver function. These results are normally back in a few days.

Other tests may include a brain-wave trace (electroencephalogram or EEG). This involves wearing something like a swimming cap with lots of wires coming off it. These traces can sometimes help distinguish different types of dementia but are not done often.

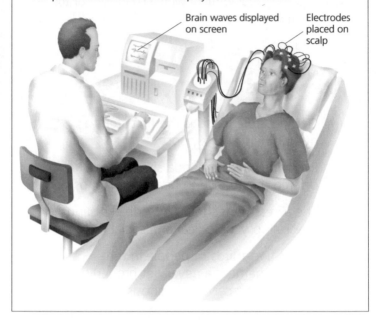

Electroencephalography (EEG)

By attaching small electrodes to the patient's scalp, a doctor can use an electroencephalography machine to monitor brain activity. The patient's brain waves are displayed on the screen.

Brain waves displayed on screen

Electrodes placed on scalp

Discussing the results of tests

When the tests are finished the specialist should sit down and be prepared to discuss the diagnosis with the person. It may be helpful to have a friend or family member there.

The doctor should ask whether the person wants to hear the diagnosis and, if he or she does, should explain this clearly and simply. This is a good opportunity also to discuss treatments, what help may be needed, and what practical, emotional and financial support is available. It is also helpful to discuss plans for the future such as appointing welfare attorneys and writing advance decisions.

It is usually difficult to take everything in at one go so a follow-up appointment with a counsellor or the doctor can be helpful.

KEY POINTS

- Getting a diagnosis is the first step to getting help and support

- Everyone with dementia should be offered the chance to hear the diagnosis

- The assessment should include checking physical, psychological and social factors

- About two-thirds of people in the UK with dementia never get properly assessed or receive a diagnosis

Treatments for dementia

Can dementia be treated?

It is important to emphasise that the mainstay of dementia care is not about drug treatment. Providing practical and emotional support, advocacy and information to the individual with dementia and their carers and family is a huge part of dementia treatment.

It is often thought that dementia cannot be treated. It is true that it cannot be cured, but there is a great deal that can be done to help. This is the focus of this chapter and the next.

Case study – Joyce

My name is Joyce and I have been getting more forgetful for three years. At first, I put this down to getting old but, when I began to lose the thread of conversations and got lost returning from the local shops, I talked to my husband Eric and we decided to get help. I went with my husband to our GP who referred me to the local hospital.

After tests confirmed I probably had Alzheimer's disease, the consultant started me on an anti-dementia drug. After three months on the medicine, I felt more confident in talking to my husband and able to go to the shops on my own again.

This chapter explains the treatments that are available for dementia including treatments for memory and challenging behaviour.

Preventing dementia

There has been very little research on what we can do to prevent getting dementia. Certain characteristics are associated with an increased risk of getting dementia. These include:

- Getting older

- Having a family history of dementia

- Head injury

- Having depression

- Drinking excessive alcohol.

Having risk factors for heart disease such as high blood pressure, diabetes, smoking, being overweight and not exercising also seem to increase the risk of getting dementia.

Except for getting older and having a strong family history, none of these risk factors has a strong link with dementia and scientists often disagree on what risks are important.

Some scientists have suggested that taking aspirin, antioxidants such as vitamin E or cholesterol-lowering drugs called statins may reduce the chance of getting dementia, but this needs further investigation.

It also seems that people who keep their brains active may be at less risk of developing dementia. Reading, engaging in a hobby such as playing bridge or chess, or doing crosswords and word puzzles may help reduce the risk.

Perhaps the best advice is to:

- Exercise the body regularly

- Exercise the brain regularly

- Keep to a healthy diet

- Drink alcohol sensibly

- Don't smoke

- Have regular check-ups to exclude diabetes and high blood pressure.

Treating dementia

There are two sets of symptoms that may need treatment in dementia. The first is the treatment of cognitive symptoms (memory loss, problems with thinking and confusion).

The second is the treatment of behavioural and psychological symptoms of dementia such as depression, anxiety, hallucinations, and irritable or aggressive behaviour, which tend to occur later in the condition.

There are frequent and often wildly exaggerated claims for new treatments in the press; these raise expectations but rarely fulfil their promise.

Treatment of memory loss and other cognitive symptoms

Until about 15 years ago there were virtually no useful drug treatments for cognitive symptoms of dementia. Now, the mainstay of treatment of memory loss in Alzheimer's disease is a group of drugs known as cholinesterase inhibitors.

There are currently three drugs in this category:

1. Donepezil (Aricept)

2. Rivastigmine (Exelon)

3. Galantamine (Reminyl).

They all work by increasing the levels of a chemical transmitter in the brain called acetylcholine (ACh). The theory is that, by boosting this chemical, nerve cells involved in memory should be able to communicate better with each other.

Some people have a definite improvement in their memory and thinking after taking these drugs, although others seem to have no benefit. Unfortunately it is not possible to predict who will and who will not benefit; the only way to tell is to try the drugs.

These medicines need to be taken every day for some weeks before an effect is likely to be seen. If one doesn't work there is probably little point in trying another. However, some people who get side effects with one drug may cope better with another in the class.

These medicines need to be started by a specialist. The doctor will probably want to check some things, including a heart trace (electrocardiogram or ECG), before starting any of these drugs.

These drugs have some side effects, although many people find them quite easy to take and don't have

How cholinesterase inhibitors work

Cholinesterase inhibitors block the activity of an enzyme in the brain that destroys the neurotransmitter acetylcholine.

1. Message transmission
Message travels along axon to synaptic knob
Neurotransmitter crosses synapse
Receptor cells are activated
Message passed on

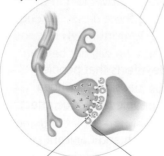

Synaptic knob

Neurotransmitter (acetylcholine)

Axon

Vesicles

Synapse

Acetylcholine reabsorbed

Cholinesterase enzyme

More acetylcholine is reabsorbed

2. After message transmission
Acetylcholine is either reabsorbed into the synaptic knob or destroyed by the enzyme cholinesterase in the synapse

3. With cholinesterase inhibition
Cholinesterase inhibitors inhibit the cholinesterase enzyme from breaking down acetylcholine, increasing both the level and duration of action of the neurotransmitter acetylcholine.

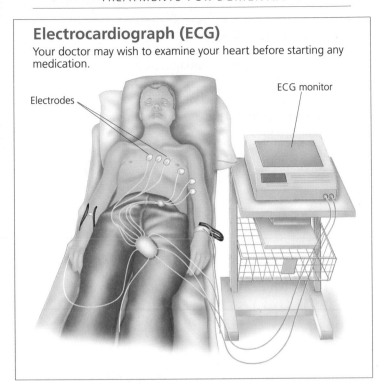

Electrocardiograph (ECG)

Your doctor may wish to examine your heart before starting any medication.

ECG monitor

Electrodes

any side effects. The main side effects that people may experience are feeling sick (nausea), diarrhoea and stomach pains. For many people these side effects improve in a few days.

The National Institute for Health and Clinical Excellence (NICE) has issued guidance on using anti-dementia drugs (see box on page 56). Recent changes in the advice have introduced more flexibility about the use of these drugs.

The current anti-dementia drugs do not stop the disease from progressing nor do they make people completely better. For someone who is responding

NICE guidance on treatment of dementia

Patients receiving anti-dementia medication should:

- Have Alzheimer's disease only

- Have a diagnosis and initial prescription by a specialist

- Be recommended acetylcholinesterase inhibitors (ACHIs) in the mild-to-moderate phase of the illness

- Be recommended memantine if they have moderate Alzheimer's disease and cannot take an ACHI or have severe dementia

- Have treatment reviewed regularly and continued while it has a worthwhile effect

to treatment it may make the difference between, say, being able and not being able to cook meals or remember to pay bills. In other words some people may be able to stay independent for longer.

After taking the tablets for between three and six months the doctor should check whether they are helping. Between one in three and one in four people who take these medicines has a definite benefit and would benefit from staying on them.

Deciding whether the medicine is helping can be difficult and the doctor will want to hear views from the patient and family/friends about the medicine.

Many other medicines have been suggested for the treatment of cognitive symptoms of dementia, but few have proved useful. Those that may help include the following.

Memantine
This drug acts on another memory chemical in the brain called NMDA (*N*-methyl-D-aspartate). It is sometimes used in moderate dementia to improve the ability to do day-to-day tasks when someone cannot tolerate acetylcholinesterase inhibitors. It may also be prescribed for the treatment of later stages of dementia.

Aspirin
Aspirin and other non-steroidal anti-inflammatory drugs have been suggested but there is insufficient research to be certain whether these are helpful.

Statins
A group of drugs used to treat high cholesterol may help prevent dementia from starting but it is unclear whether they improve symptoms if dementia has already started.

Ginkgo biloba
Ginkgo biloba, a widely used plant extract, has been the subject of numerous clinical trials. Unfortunately, it appears to have only a modest effect on dementia.

Treatment of behavioural symptoms
Case study – Richard
Richard lived with his partner, Andrew, in a basement flat. Richard had developed dementia about four years ago. Now, Richard was becoming a bit of a handful; he was incontinent of urine and most afternoons got quite

agitated, trying to get out of the flat and shouting that he wanted to go home. He did not recognise that the flat was his home!

Andrew was very keen to care for Richard at home, but was finding it increasingly difficult. The local hospital sent a community nurse who specialised in dementia. She gave Andrew advice about how to deal with Richard's incontinence, including taking him to the toilet regularly and using special pads.

The nurse also suggested that, instead of trying to keep Richard in the flat in the afternoon, as soon as he became agitated, Andrew should take him for a walk around the block. When he did this, Richard was much more settled in the evenings.

When Alois Alzheimer first described Alzheimer's disease, he noted that some of the most difficult symptoms were not to do with memory but changes in mood and behaviour. Nearly all people with dementia will experience some changes in behaviour or mood. These are shown in the table opposite.

Many of these symptoms can cause a great deal of distress for people with dementia and those caring for them. Some, such as depression, can make the memory problems worse and may reduce the ability to do everyday tasks.

Sometimes a physical reason, such as a urine infection or constipation, is the cause of the symptoms. For these reasons anyone showing any of these symptoms should be seen by a doctor to exclude a physical cause. Once a physical cause has been ruled out, the treatment depends on the symptom.

It is helpful to see these symptoms in the context of the person, and the past and current environment.

Changes in behaviour or mood that are common in Alzheimer's disease

Very common	Common	Less common
Apathy	Agitation	Crying
Verbal or physical aggression	Disinhibition	Mannerisms (repeated actions)
Wandering and restlessness	Screaming	Delusions
Eating problems	Sexual problems	Hallucinations (seeing or hearing things that are not there)
Sleeping problems		
Depression		
Anxiety		
Repeated questioning		

To enable this a 'life story' can be extremely helpful. A life story builds up a profile of the person, his or her background, education, hobbies and career, relationships and personality characteristics.

Building a life story can be very useful if someone enters a care home, as the staff caring for the person will have a far better understanding of the person. Often staff will create a life story with the help of the person with dementia and his or her family and friends. This can take the form of an album, with photographs.

Case study – Alice
Music was Alice's first and greatest love. She had been in various choirs since the age of eight. She was an accomplished pianist and also played the flute. She worked as a volunteer for many years teaching music in the local prison. She had a huge collection of classical music records.

Alice had Alzheimer's disease for eight years and had recently moved into a residential home. Although she visited the home before moving in, and seemed to like it, once there she became increasingly anxious, depressed and irritable.

She would pace around the corridors and sometimes shout out if she was sat in front of the television. The staff in the home were aware of Alice's life story and thought that she was upset because she had been deprived of her music. Her grandson came to the rescue; he bought an MP3 player and put a lot of her music onto it. Alice now listens to her music frequently and seems more content.

If depression is severe, it should probably be treated with antidepressant tablets because depression can make the symptoms of dementia so much worse. For many other symptoms the treatment should start with non-drug approaches. The approach should be decided after carefully analysing the symptoms.

Agitation and restlessness
Repetitive purposeless movements and pacing around may be the result of pain or discomfort or a sign of boredom, but often just happen with no explanation. These are some of the most distressing symptoms for the carer but sometimes do not appear to be distressing for the person with dementia.

If not too extreme the best thing may be just to tolerate the restlessness. However, sometimes adjusting the routine (as in the example of Richard, page 57) may help to reduce the problem.

In the past these problems were often treated using sedative drugs, but these drugs have been found to be harmful in some people with dementia (they may cause falls, excessive sedation or stroke) and should be used only in the most extreme situations when prescribed by a specialist.

Analysing the behaviour to find out the causes and consequences may help find the solution, as shown in the next case.

Case study – James

James was a big man – well over 6 feet tall. He cut quite a striking figure in the nursing home where he lived. James had vascular dementia which affected his speech, and one of his major problems was that he found it very difficult to make himself understood.

Over some weeks James became more aggressive, sometimes hitting staff or other residents. The staff at the home were at the end of their tether and demanded that James be moved to hospital.

An analysis of this behaviour showed that most of James' aggression took place around meal times. The nurse observed that when the food was being served James became increasingly agitated and sometimes aggressive, and that the longer James had to wait for his food the worse things became.

Also, it seemed as if James was still hungry after the meal (he was receiving the same size portions as all the other residents). They decided to try giving James his food first and to give him an extra helping; this worked like a dream. The aggression subsided and James was able to continue living in the home.

Eating problems

People with dementia experience changes in taste for food and appetite. Many people lose weight once they develop dementia, despite getting more of a taste for sweet foods. A more flexible approach to meals – possibly serving finger food or smaller meals more often, and changing the diet to suit the individual – can help.

Sleeping problems

Not being able to sleep at night is a common difficulty. People may get up in the early hours and think it is daytime; they may get dressed and try to go to work. Sleep problems at night are often made worse by napping during the day and lack of exercise.

The first step should be getting into a routine with exercise and fresh air every day, avoiding 'cat naps', and avoiding heavy meals or stimulating drinks (such as coffee) before bedtime. Thick curtains may help stop someone waking early, and a clock by the bed may help remind them it's night-time.

Anxiety and depression

These often go hand in hand and are common in dementia. Depression can make many symptoms of dementia, such as forgetfulness, poor concentration and lack of motivation, even worse.

If someone with dementia is suspected of having depression he or she should be seen by a doctor urgently because he or she may need antidepressants (tablets that help depression).

Crying

Crying can occur even if someone does not seem depressed. Sometimes people just go from being happy to crying and back to happy like flicking a switch. This is called emotional lability. It is often upsetting for onlookers but the person with lability may not appear distressed. Sometimes antidepressants can help.

Disinhibition

Disinhibition is the loss of usual control over our impulses. For example, if we see a very attractive person we may have the desire to kiss them, but stop ourselves from doing this.

Disinhibition can be one of the most difficult symptoms to cope with. People may say cutting or hurtful things or behave inappropriately – for example, urinating in public, or making sexual suggestions to family, friends or passers-by. These can be difficult to treat and may require a specialist opinion. Sometimes, in extreme cases, sedatives may be needed to reduce the behaviour.

Sexual problems

Sexual problems, such as excessive demands for sex, masturbating in public, touching the genitalia or making sexual demands on strangers, can be very embarrassing and upsetting for partners and carers.

It has to be remembered at all times that this behaviour is due to the disease not the person. It can be equally upsetting if a person no longer wants to have sex and the partner feels very rejected. If any of these problems occur, it can be helpful to talk things over with a specialist nurse or doctor who can often make helpful suggestions. Sometimes drugs can be used to reduce sex drive.

Equally frustrating (for a partner) can be a loss of sex drive that may accompany dementia. Libido will vary over time, but persistent loss of sexual relations can happen. Trying different ways to rekindle a partner's interest in sex (if this is what they want) may help.

Delusions and hallucinations

Delusions (the person believing that someone is stealing things or trying to harm him or her) and hallucinations (seeing or hearing things that are not there) are often seen in people with dementia.

If these are not causing distress, it may be best to leave them alone. A group of drugs called antipsychotics (normally used in the treatment of schizophrenia) may help reduce these symptoms but should be prescribed only by a specialist who reviews the person regularly.

Changing pattern of symptoms

Whatever the cause of dementia the behavioural and psychological symptoms are likely to change in type and severity as the dementia progresses. For this reason, people should have their treatment reviewed regularly.

KEY POINTS

■ Keeping your body healthy and brain active may help to prevent dementia

■ Memory loss and other cognitive symptoms may be helped by treatment with anti-dementia drugs called cholinesterase inhibitors

■ Behavioural symptoms should be seen in the context of the life story – sedative drugs should be given only as a last resort

Getting help

How to get help – who pays?

Help is available from a variety of sources and all the professionals listed below may be useful. Any person with dementia and his or her carer are entitled to a needs assessment, which is normally carried out by a social worker or an occupational therapist from the local social services department.

This assessment is free but you may have to ask for it. You can ring the local social services department or your GP may be able to put you in touch. The assessment may reveal a number of needs for which help is required.

A named key worker, usually the social worker, will draw up a care plan and discuss your needs and tell you what is available locally. The sorts of help available may include home care (for help with shopping and cleaning), help with personal care (washing and dressing), meals on wheels, day care and respite. This help is usually means tested so you may have to pay for it yourself or make a contribution to the cost.

They use criteria called 'fair access to services'. There are four bands of need: low, moderate, substantial and critical. Some authorities only help pay for people judged to have substantial or critical needs. Depending on what band you are in you may have to pay for, or contribute to, care that you need.

Local authorities are increasingly using a process called 'personal budget'. This is an allocation of funding paid to someone so that they can arrange for the help that they need themselves (with the help of their family if necessary). Personal budgets give the person more flexibility and control, but arranging and supervising care can be stressful.

If you are asked to pay for help and you feel that this is unfair or you cannot afford it, check with the Alzheimer's Society helpline or the local Citizens Advice Bureau.

Types of help

All people with dementia and their carers will need help. The types of assistance most frequently needed are:

- Information

- Practical help

- Medical help

- Personal support.

Support and services for people with dementia varies widely around the country – in some areas they may be very good, in others they may be limited. The National Dementia Strategy in England, and similar developments in other countries, will hopefully ensure that good services are more widely available.

Information

Information is going to be needed on all aspects of dementia, and on where to find help. Most information can be obtained free but you might want to buy one or two books. The information required will change as time goes on.

Many financial benefits are available for people with dementia and their carers, and advice on these, together with advice on arranging a will or a lasting power of attorney, are all matters about which information will be needed.

There are a large number of sources of help. Your local GP is a good place to start because he or she should know what services exist locally.

Many local boroughs have dementia support teams. The Alzheimer's Society can provide a great deal of information that is well written and easy to understand. Many areas have Alzheimer's Society support groups.

Other voluntary organisations such as the Pick's Disease Support Group and Lewy Body Society can provide information. Admiral Nurses (nurses attached to local health providers but trained by a charity called Dementia UK) can provide help, advocacy and practical support to carers of people with dementia.

There are now several books for people with dementia and their carers. See 'Useful information' (page 126) for contact details.

Practical help

The need for help in the home and adaptations to the home is going to change as time goes on. This is why it is so important that the carer's needs assessment is done and that a social worker takes responsibility for ensuring that the needs are met and reassessed from time to time. The needs in the home may include the following:

- Help in the home with the housework, shopping, meals on wheels

- Safety aids and equipment such as commodes, a laundry service, advice on moving and handling, special clothing, hoists

- Home security: a recent development known as assistive technology, or telecare, can provide imaginative aids to help make the home more safe and secure; these include alarms triggered if a front door is opened or someone falls over, and sensors that sound an alarm if the taps or gas is left on

- Help with bathing, getting up in the morning, dressing and going to bed at night.

Medical help

Regular visits to the doctor for both the person with dementia and separately for the carer are important. The person with dementia needs:

- Checks with his or her doctor on a regular basis, ideally every six months

- Prompt treatment for other health problems such as depression or infections that might occur

- General health advice about diet and exercise

- Advice on behavioural changes for the carer to be able to understand and manage

- Regular foot care, checks of vision and hearing, and visits to the dentist.

The carer needs to care for his or her own health also. A healthy, cheerful carer will make a big difference to the person with dementia with whom they are living or to whom they are close.

Personal support

There are several ways in which both the carer and the person with dementia can receive personal support. The social worker who is responsible for following up the needs assessment referred to above can arrange the following.

Taking a break/respite care

Looking after someone with dementia and being looked after can both be emotionally draining. Struggling to manage on one's own can be self-defeating and can make life for the person with dementia more difficult.

It is usually important that both the person with dementia and the carer have time apart. It is therefore very important for there to be breaks in caring and being cared for. The carer will benefit by being able to socialise with friends, pursue interests or just spend time in the home without having to supervise the person with dementia.

The person with dementia will benefit from being able to socialise with other people and take part in other activities.

Respite can take various forms. The person with dementia might be able to attend a day centre one or more days of the week if it is available locally and he or she is willing.

It might be possible for someone to come into the home to be with the person with dementia while the carer goes out for an afternoon or evening. Social

services may be able to offer longer respite breaks
(usually a week or two) in a care home.

Someone to talk to

Both carers and people with dementia have described
the benefits of talking to other people with similar
problems. Support groups exist in all parts of the country
that meet regularly. Information about what is available
locally can be obtained from your social worker or by
contacting the Alzheimer's Society or Age UK.

Permanent residential and nursing care

There may come a time when caring for a person with
dementia in his or her own home is getting too difficult
or no longer possible. This will involve discussion
among the person with dementia, the carer, the GP or
hospital specialist, and the social worker. This might
arise if the person with dementia is living alone and
becoming a risk to her- or himself because it is rarely
possible to provide 24-hour care to a single person at
home except at great expense.

It might arise if the carer living with the person with
dementia is physically and/or mentally frail and cannot
manage even with daily help and respite care.

There are three main types of care setting: extra care
shelter (such as sheltered housing but with 24-hour
care available), residential homes and nursing homes.
A social worker will assess someone for funding if they
are thought to need permanent residential care and all
options of keeping someone at home have been tried.

Who can help?

Health and social services

The person with dementia, the carer and the social

worker together with the GP coordinate the care throughout the illness. The GP will be the main person to look after the health care of the person with dementia and the carer.

For a firm diagnosis to be made and advice to be given on further treatment and management, the GP will often refer the person with dementia and the carer to a specialist. This is a free service.

The specialist might be:

- An old age psychiatrist (a doctor specialising in the mental disorders of old age)

- A neurologist (a specialist in diseases of the nervous system)

- A geriatrician (a specialist in medical diseases of older people).

Exactly which specialist someone is referred to will depend on:

- Their age

- What symptoms they have

- What services are available locally.

Sometimes it may be necessary for a person to see more than one specialist; for example, a neurologist may ask an old age psychiatrist for a second opinion if symptoms of depression are present.

If the specialist is the old age psychiatrist he or she will be part of a community mental health team that often includes social workers, psychologists, occupational therapists and specialist nurses. As the illness progresses free support and advice may be given by one or more of the members of this team. The other specialists do not generally have a back-up team.

This team or the GP can refer to social services for help with bathing and dressing, to the podiatrist/ chiropodist for foot care or to the continence adviser.

The occupational therapist can advise on ways of helping someone to maintain their skills and independence for as long as possible. They can also advise on aids in the person's home.

The social worker can organise breaks/respite from caring or being cared for. This can be provided by a number of different agencies – voluntary, private or state – and might have to be paid for.

The social worker will discuss with the person with dementia and the carer what might be most helpful and as time goes on these needs might change.

There are a number of possibilities adapted to the particular needs of the person with dementia and the carer, changing with time and local availability and which might have to be paid for. These are:

- Sitters at home to allow a carer to go out for a few hours, an evening, a weekend.

- Paid carers or volunteers to go out with a person with dementia.

- Day care organised either by social services or by a voluntary organisation such as the Alzheimer's Society or Age UK, depending on what is available locally. A person with dementia should be able to go for an agreed number of days a week. Transport is usually arranged by the agency running the day centre.

The professionals involved in care

The various professionals who may help in dementia care are shown below. As many people now work in teams, these roles are not so clear cut.

Professional	Role
General practitioner (GP)	Referring for diagnosis, medical care
Psychiatrist	Diagnosis, starting and monitoring treatment
Neurologist	Diagnosis, rare kinds of dementia
Occupational therapist	Enhancing function; making environment safe, assessment for assistive technology
Community nurse	Monitoring progress and treatment, counselling
Admiral nurse	Counselling and support for carers
Social worker	Organising benefits, home care, respite, care homes, support
Psychologist	Specialist memory tests; analysing behaviour
Speech and language therapist	Improving communication, swallowing problems

- Short-term residential care for a weekend or one or more weeks to allow a carer to go on holiday or just have time on his or her own at home. This can be provided by social services or by the voluntary or private sector, depending on what is available locally.

- Permanent residential or nursing home care: this can be arranged with the help of a social worker if the criteria for residential care are met. It is advisable to look at a number of homes. Choice will depend on an assessment of the person with dementia and matching the needs of the person with those that can be met by the home.

The Alzheimer's Society (www.alzheimers.org.uk)

The Alzheimer's Society is dedicated to supporting people with all types of dementias and their families and provides:

- Information on all the dementias

- Practical and emotional help such as helplines and support groups

- Legal and financial advice

- Training for carers

- Services such as respite care.

Going online – www.alzheimers.org.uk – is one of the easiest ways of obtaining information. However, if either the person with dementia or the carer has an urgent question, they are strongly advised to telephone the Alzheimer's Society national helpline on 0845 300 0336.

An online forum called Talking Point at www. alzheimers.org.uk/talkingpoint/site/index.php can be accessed on the Alzheimer's Society website. This is available 24/7 and allows you to ask questions, respond to queries from others and participate in discussion (see 'Useful information', page 127).

Joining the Alzheimer's Society (see 'Useful information', page 127) and receiving the newsletter help people to keep in touch with news and practical advice.

Other voluntary organisations and social services, which provide information, include:

- Carers UK

- The Princess Royal Trust for Carers

- Dementia UK (a charity that supports Admiral Nurses)

- Age UK

- Citizens Advice – can provide free advice on benefits

- Local social services department.

You can find their contact details at the end of this book.

KEY POINTS

- People with dementia, and people who look after them, will need information, practical help, medical care and personal support; don't go it alone

- Every carer is entitled to a free needs assessment from the local social services department; ask for it

- Use the Alzheimer's Society; it is there to help you

Living with dementia: tips for people with dementia and for carers

Tips for the person with dementia

Over the last ten years more people with dementia have been diagnosed earlier. This has meant that it has been possible to talk to people in the early stages and learn from them what it is like to have the condition.

Not so long ago it was thought impossible that people with dementia could contribute to an understanding of their predicament. Now we have learnt a whole range of emotional reactions that they experience from them.

They may be angry: 'Why me?' They may be fearful: 'How will I cope?' 'How will my family cope?' They may feel sad and despairing: 'What is the point of going on?' They may feel alone.

General tips

Here are some tips for people with dementia from people with dementia themselves: if your memory is not as good as it used to be you might find it helpful to:

- Keep a diary

- Hang a white board in the kitchen with your weekly timetable and reminders of things that you need to do

- Put labels on doors and drawers to remind you where things are kept

- Keep a list of telephone numbers with names by the phone

- Have a newspaper delivered each day; reading this will help to keep your brain active and remind you of the date

- Put things like keys always in the same place to increase the chance of finding them each time that you look for them

- Tell your family that you do not mind being reminded about things that you need to know.

Try to keep cheerful and not get depressed. Talk to your friends and family. Stay as active as possible. Keep up your interests and your friends. Don't be afraid to ask for support. Join a group of other people with dementia, which the Alzheimer's Society can find for you. Sharing feelings and ideas with other people with dementia can be very supportive. You might also want to help the Alzheimer's Society in their work.

At work

If the diagnosis of dementia has been made and you are still at work, unless you are self-employed, you will probably feel that you should leave your job. You or your employer may agree that it is reasonable for you to continue working. You may be pleasantly surprised how considerate people are if they are involved early on.

It might be possible for you to work fewer hours or stay but in a different role. You need to ensure that people do tell you if you are not coping and you need to feel able to ask for support when you need it.

At the point that you stop working make sure that you have secured your full pension rights and also get advice about any benefits to which you might be entitled as early as possible, while you are still able to understand them. If your employer has a human resources department there will be someone to help you. If this is not the case try the Citizens Advice Bureau.

Make sure that you make out a lasting power of attorney so that your affairs can be dealt with if and when you can no longer take responsibility yourself (see below). When you do stop working try to make sure that you find things to occupy you. Keeping busy, involved and interested is important.

Driving

Dementia can affect people's ability to drive safely. They may feel that they are able to get about on familiar routes without incident. The problem is that, when a hazard arises, the person may not be able to react as quickly or as well as someone without dementia.

Having a diagnosis of dementia does not mean an automatic driving ban. The person must tell the Driver and Vehicle Licensing Agency (DVLA) and insurance company when he or she is diagnosed with dementia.

The person is advised not to drive while waiting for the decision from the DVLA. The DVLA may then seek a medical report from the doctor, and may decide to allow the person to continue driving, or offer another driving test.

Sometimes the DVLA will revoke the driving licence. It is not possible to hold a LGV (Large Goods Vehicle) licence or PCV (Public Carriage Vehicle) licence if you have dementia. It is important to be open and honest with the DVLA and the insurance company.

Use of public transport or taxis and walking are probably all safer alternatives.

Everyone has a responsibility to avoid harm not just to themselves but also to the general public. Driving ability usually deteriorates in the 70s and 80s anyway, but this is much more the case in people with dementia so our advice is to consider stopping driving once you have been given a definite diagnosis of dementia.

Financial affairs
General advice
You might need to consult a solicitor about some of the things mentioned below. Make paying bills as simple as possible by getting these paid through the bank on standing orders. Setting up a joint account with a partner may make day-to-day money management easier.

Make sure that you receive all the benefits to which you are entitled. You will be able to obtain this information through the Alzheimer's Society helpline (see 'Useful information', page 127).

Make a will

Most people in the UK don't have a will. Dying intestate (without a will) can cause problems for the bereaved family and may mean that assets are left to the wrong people. Writing a will is usually straightforward.

It is probably best to consult a solicitor if you have already been given a diagnosis of dementia. It is still possible for someone with dementia to write a valid will provided that he or she has 'testamentary capacity'. This means that the person knows the purpose of a will, can name people who may have a claim on the estate and know (roughly) how much his or her estate is worth.

Making decisions

As dementia progresses people are less able to make decisions for themselves. However, in the early stages, many people can make these decisions and influence their lives and care later on.

To be able to make decisions about care, people must have 'capacity'. This means that they can understand and retain information given to them about the issue being decided (for example, a course of treatment or move to a residential home) and the alternative ways of dealing with that issue, weigh this information in the balance and tell someone what they have decided.

If you don't have capacity, people caring for you (doctors, nurses, social workers, etc.) will have to make decisions on your behalf. This is why it is important to set up an advance decision or appoint a power of attorney while you are able to.

A lasting power of attorney (welfare attorney and/or financial attorney, see page 84) can be completed only if someone has capacity to do this. This is the best way of ensuring that decisions can be made for you, and enable someone you trust to look after your finances for you and/or oversee your personal and social care should the time come that you are not able to do this.

If you have not appointed a welfare attorney (see page 84), a relative should be consulted about major decisions about care (for example, going into a nursing home).

If there is no one who can do this for you, your social worker will organise for you to have an independent mental capacity advocate (IMCA).

IMCAs are there to help if a serious decision, such as moving into residential care, needs to be made for you. The IMCA is an independent person who has completed IMCA training and has a background of relevant experience. The role of the IMCA is to support and represent the needs of the person with dementia and do his or her best to ensure that the right decision is made on that person's behalf.

Advance decisions on treatment

An advance decision allows you to state what treatments you do not wish to receive. It also allows you to communicate your views on issues such as the sanctity of life.

You cannot compel doctors to give a specific treatment in an advance decision but you can give guidance about the types of treatment that you would want to have or avoid.

A suggested form to make out an advance decision can be obtained from the Alzheimer's Society. It is important to give a copy to your GP and to your close family, friends or next of kin.

Lasting power of attorney (LPA)

There are two types of lasting power of attorney (LPA):

1. Financial

2. Welfare.

These need to be set up separately. Although the forms are available from the internet or the Office of the Public Guardian (see page 132) they are quite complicated. You might want to get the help of a solicitor even though this makes it more expensive. 'Solicitors for the Elderly' (see page 134) may be helpful in finding a solicitor in your area.

Financial LPA

A financial LPA gives power to someone whom you nominate to run finances such as writing cheques, making investments, etc.

Welfare LPA

A welfare LPA gives power to someone whom you choose to make decisions about your medical and social care on your behalf. You can appoint the same person as both financial and welfare attorneys.

You can appoint more than one attorney if you wish and the welfare attorney and finance attorney can be different people. When completing the form you can make statements on what you would like to happen (or not happen). When you complete the forms an independent person (either someone who knows you well or a professional such as a doctor) needs to sign the application stating that you have capacity and are completing the form voluntarily.

Tips for the carer

Mrs X, who looks after her husband, says it all:

'My husband first showed symptoms of dementia some years ago. My great difficulty then was getting the professionals to LISTEN to me – he presented so well, and was very good at "covering up".

'Now, I know that my quality of life is important and is directly linked with my husband's. When I am exhausted, depressed, emotionally drained, suppressing my irritation and not being able to respond in the usual way to verbal abuse and false accusations, I find it very difficult to be patient, tolerant and understanding.

'I now am very fortunate as my husband goes in for respite care every six weeks for one to two weeks, and this gives me the chance to sleep, relax and do the things I am unable to do as a result of my husband's condition.

'He has changed from a confident, capable, outgoing person to become a nervous, frightened, agitated man who no longer reads, enjoys television or socialises, and scarcely allows me out of his sight.'

Life for the carer can be exhausting. People with dementia have increasing difficulty carrying out the activities of daily living without support from their carers. Life seems to slow down because everything takes so much longer.

People with dementia may not want to be helped with some of the more private tasks and may become very difficult without being able to explain why.

Behaviour can become an embarrassment so that the carer is ashamed to invite friends home or to go out with the person. This means that carers are in danger of becoming isolated and lonely.

The person with dementia might sleep poorly and get mixed up between day and night, with the result that the carer gets very tired. The carer may get very sad that he or she has lost the person whom he or she knew.

All these emotions can make carers depressed, angry and irritable, and react impatiently and aggressively to the person with whom they are living and for whom they are caring.

This can make the carers feel guilty and even more so if occasionally they feel that they can no longer cope and want to put the person with dementia into a home.

Carers may worry about all the financial implications of caring for someone with a chronic illness.

All these emotions are bound to occur to a lesser or greater extent but they can be substantially reduced with the appropriate advice, information and support. Living with and caring for a person with dementia are challenging.

Here are some general guidelines and tips for carers that other carers have found helpful.

Tips on dealing with toileting and incontinence

The person with dementia may lose the ability to recognise when to go to the toilet, where the toilet is or what to do when in the toilet. The following are some suggestions that other carers have found helpful:

- Remind the person to go to the toilet at regular intervals and always before bedtime or before going out

- Make sure that the toilet is easy to find, well lit and warm, and leave the door open

- Make sure that clothing is easy to remove

- Limit drinks before bedtime or before going out

- Provide a bottle/commode by the bed side

- Ask advice from the GP who will put you in touch
  with a continence adviser who might be helpful
  about use of pads and waterproof covers for the
  chair and bed.

Tips on dealing with washing and bathing
The person with dementia may forget to wash and no
longer recognise the need. Here are some tips:

- Try to establish and maintain a routine

- Make it fun

- Respect the person's dignity

- Think about safety

- If it is a constant problem ask the GP to refer you
  for help from the district nursing service.

**Understand what is happening to the person
being cared for**

- People with loss of memory are going to find it
  difficult to understand what is going on around
  them, where they are and whom they are with.

- They might have difficult expressing themselves or
  understanding what is being said.

- They may be frustrated that they cannot do things
  for themselves and become very resistant.

- Their behaviour might vary from day to day and sometimes within a day. This is the nature of the illness.

It is important for the carer to understand and try to remember that these difficulties are part of the brain disease and not the fault of the person with dementia.

Try to find out as much as possible about dementia and how it is affecting the person for whom you are caring. Your personal knowledge of the person with dementia will often mean that you can understand why he or she is behaving in the way that he or she is when this is impossible or at least difficult for professionals.

Keep things normal

Try to keep life going as it has always has been for as long as possible. Having a daily routine is helpful but there is a need to be flexible. Keep doing all the things that you have always enjoyed together and seeing friends and family.

Try to consult and involve the person in all decisions, large or small, at all times. This will ensure that his or her self-esteem is maintained for as long as possible.

Retain the person's independence

It is important that people with dementia continue to carry out the tasks of which they are capable for as long as possible. Everything might take longer and sometimes they may need prompting.

It is often helpful to simplify the tasks, for example laying the clothes on the bed in such a way that the person is assisted to remember in what order to put them on. This allows the person affected to retain a sense of person and dignity.

Encourage activities that a person with dementia has always been interested in doing but remember that with the progression of the illness these interests might change, and you need to pick this up early so as not to cause upset.

Avoid confrontation

Try not to argue when, for example, a person can see no reason for having a bath or changing clothes, or accuses you or someone else of taking his or her money when he or she cannot find something. Walk away briefly or think of a distraction and try later.

Avoid crises

When planning to go out leave enough time so that there is no rush. Remember that unfamiliar places and people will be very confusing. Prepare for these situations by talking and going over things many times beforehand.

Try to anticipate what might happen from what you have already learnt. You are the expert because you know the person for whom you are caring better than anyone else.

Try to have a laugh

Life is not easy but the more relaxed you are the better. If you can have a laugh with the person for whom you are caring you will both find it easier to cope.

Lots of hugs can be very reassuring provided, of course, that the person for whom you are caring finds this acceptable.

Make sure that your home is as safe as possible

A confused person is more at risk of accidents simply because he or she is not paying enough attention through problems with concentration.

Try to ensure that there are no loose rugs or mats around and that there are handrails up the stairs and in the bathroom. Make sure that slippers fit snugly to reduce the likelihood of falls.

Gas needs to be switched off at the mains if you go out and leave the person for whom you are caring alone. Don't leave matches around.

General health

Regular exercise such as a daily walk and a good diet are essential. The longer the person is fully mobile and physically healthy and cheerful the easier for you and therefore for him or her.

Take particular care over any drugs taken, supervise them and try to know what each drug is for. Question the doctor if you are not sure about any aspect of medication and if they do not appear to be having any effect. Ask whether any of the drugs can be stopped – the fewer drugs the better.

Make sure that you arrange for the person for whom you are caring to have regular checks of vision, hearing, feet and teeth.

Make meal times pleasurable

We all enjoy eating and drinking. Try to involve the person with whom you are living in the planning and preparing of meals and then allowing enough time to enjoy it together with a glass of beer or wine, if that is what you have always enjoyed.

Remembering the types of food that the person always used to enjoy can he helpful in deciding what would give most pleasure.

It is important to try to encourage the person to be as independent as possible so, when the person has difficulty with cutlery, you should offer finger foods more often.

Communication with the person with dementia

Try to gain the person's attention before speaking and remember to speak slowly, clearly and at eye level. Listen and observe carefully. Be prepared to repeat things many times.

Remember that your body language also conveys how you are feeling and will be picked up by the person for whom you are caring.

Telling children and grandchildren about the person with dementia

It is important that children and grandchildren understand about dementia and learn to accept that this is an illness and that they can still give a great deal of pleasure to their parent or grandparent. If children are at school, they will then be able to talk about it to their teachers and friends, and this will mean that they do not, for example, feel embarrassed when inviting friends home.

Memory aids

It is helpful to write important things down, for example plans for the day on a calendar or board in a place that is frequently used. This is useful for things such as plans for the day, or remembering names of people who might be visiting. It is useful to have telephone numbers and names of people with whom one is in regular contact near the telephone. In addition:

- Have a clock with clear numbers

- Label doors

- Have photos of family members around

- When visitors or family come repeatedly mention their names and who they are.

Communication with the doctor

A good and positive relationship with your doctor and members of the mental health team can make all the difference to how supported you and the person for whom you are caring feel. This will mean working out how best to achieve it.

Going to the doctor on a regular basis is important. It does not need to be often. Making the next appointment after each visit is a good idea. It is helpful to come to each visit with some prepared notes on, for example, the patient's general health, changes in the symptoms or behaviour of the person for whom you are caring, side effects of medicines, your own health (see below) and help needed.

When you visit don't be afraid to ask if you do not understand something or want the doctor to repeat something that you have been told. Take notes of what has been said and then you can go over it afterwards.

Look after your own physical and mental health

This is as important as the health of the person for whom you are caring. It is just too easy to neglect your own diet and forget to take exercise when you are busy and exhausted. It is so easy to ignore health problems of your own and not take time to go to the doctor if you need to (see 'Getting help', page 66).

KEY POINTS

- If you have dementia, try lots of different memory aids; hopefully you will find one that suits you and combats the effects of the disease

- If you care for someone with dementia, make sure that you look after your own health and needs

- There are many sources of help and support available – use them!

Future prospects

Dementia is on the increase. Currently there are about 700,000 people in the UK with various stages of dementia; this will rise to about 1 million by 2025.

The main reason for this rise is that people are living longer and people born in the baby boom years are reaching an age where dementia is likely.

In 2008, the estimated cost of dementia care in the UK was £17 billion. The bulk of this was the cost of informal (unpaid) care and accommodation.

Despite this there has been relatively little research into dementia. For every person with cancer about £300 is spent on research compared with £11 for every person with dementia.

Better diagnoses

A high proportion of people with early dementia are not seen by a doctor until they have had the condition for some time, often years rather than months. Many never receive a diagnosis.

This needs to change in the future. This can happen only if there is a further increase in public awareness and a reduction in the stigma associated with the diagnosis.

When assessing people who do come with early signs of the condition, the capacity of doctors to make an accurate diagnosis depends largely on the history from the person and his or her family or friends.

Brain scans, memory tests, brain-wave traces and other tests can help with the diagnosis but there is no definitive test for dementia.

In the early stages of dementia, it can be impossible to tell for sure whether someone actually has dementia, or just the minor memory problems that we all get with advancing age.

Developing more accurate tests, especially if they can diagnose dementia very early, is important. More accurate and earlier diagnosis will mean that people can receive treatments more quickly and have more time to maximise the quality of life.

Some people have a reversible dementia due to a treatable condition such as an underactive thyroid gland or vitamin deficiency. Although relatively rare, it is important that doctors recognise when a dementia is treatable so that the cause can be treated.

At the moment about two-thirds of people with dementia do not receive a proper diagnosis so these causes may be missed. All people who develop memory difficulties or problems with thinking should be seen by a doctor to check whether the cause is reversible.

At present doctors can reliably tell what type of dementia (for example, vascular dementia or Alzheimer's disease) a person has about 80 per cent of the time, based mainly on the history and brain scan.

As better treatments emerge for specific types of dementia, the accuracy of telling what type of dementia someone has will become very important, so better tests are needed to distinguish the causes.

New and promising developments to aid diagnosis are in the pipeline. Scientists are looking at whether blood tests or tests on the fluid surrounding the spine can help diagnose Alzheimer's disease.

New scanning techniques are being developed. One involves injecting a chemical that links on to amyloid (the chemical laid down in the brain in Alzheimer's disease) and shows up on a special brain scan called positron emission tomography (PET).

Better standards of care

Most people with dementia are looked after at home, but about a third are looked after in residential homes. If they are living at home, the quality of care that people receive will depend, as well as on a whole range of other factors, on whether their carers are well informed about the condition and its course, and on how much help and support they get from other members of the family, professionals and the local authority.

At the present time, professional help and support by local services are very variable. Carers are often poorly informed and this needs to change, so that all carers have easy access to the information that they need from the sources that we have already cited.

Many people with dementia will eventually need care in residential homes. Again the quality of such homes is currently very variable and, in some places, deplorably low.

It is vital that people who look after individuals with dementia are properly trained, valued in society and adequately rewarded, and have a career path.

Expectations of the standards of care and support for people living at home and in care homes need to rise.

The National Dementia Strategy for England, launched in 2009, will hopefully ensure that dementia care has a high priority in society. The key themes of this strategy are:

- Improving public and professional awareness

- Early diagnosis and intervention

- Improving quality of care.

In the future it is likely that much greater effort will be made to involve people with dementia in making decisions involving their care than has been the case in the past. Until very recently it has been assumed that it is not really worthwhile to try to find out what such people would like to happen, so professionals and sometimes even family members have not bothered to ask them.

With earlier diagnosis many more people with dementia are able to take part in decision-making. Indeed the 2007 Mental Capacity Act makes it compulsory for carers and professionals to consult people with dementia before decisions are taken across a whole range of situations.

Treatments and cures

Up to now, dementia has not been seen as a priority for research but that is changing. Also, because scientists have not worked out precisely what causes the many different types of dementia it is difficult to work out what may be a useful treatment.

It seems that almost every week there is some story in the press about a new 'miracle cure'. These stories are nearly always misleading. Although there are many treatments being investigated, these are mainly aimed at helping symptoms of dementia. We are probably many years away from a cure.

However, there are some promising new treatments being developed. These include drugs to improve memory and help slow down the processes underlying dementia.

Most of the current research is on Alzheimer's disease. As more is understood about how Alzheimer's disease develops scientists are developing drugs that tackle the disease at different stages.

Some of these drugs hold the promise of slowing the progression of the disease. Currently there are over 40 drugs being investigated.

Anti-amyloid drugs

Some drugs are designed to lower the levels of amyloid protein (an abnormal protein laid down in the brains of people with Alzheimer's disease) or reduce the formation of amyloid. Scientists are also investigating the possibility of immunising people against amyloid.

Tau therapies

A compound that helps brain cells keep their shape, called tau, shows abnormalities in Alzheimer's disease. As a result the brain cells change shape and die off, resulting in clumps called tangles. The death of brain cells is probably responsible for the symptoms of dementia. Drugs that reduce the abnormal type of tau have shown early promise in treating Alzheimer's disease and are being researched further.

Nerve growth factor

A third approach is to boost levels of a chemical called nerve growth factor. This is present in all brains and helps the nerve cells stay healthy. Several drugs that increase levels of nerve growth factor (including statins, which are used to treat high cholesterol) are being studied.

Research is also taking place on other compounds such as omega-3 fat (found in fish oils) and many other drugs.

The drug development process

At the moment it must seem frustrating to see all these medicines being developed, yet so few are available on prescription. This is because it takes years of study to make sure that a compound is effective and safe.

Drugs have to pass through various stages of development (phases 1, 2 and 3) before they can reach the market. Fewer than 1 in 20 drugs in development becomes licensed. However, with so much research under way, it seems likely that more effective treatments will become available.

Treatments for behaviour problems

At least as important as drug treatments for memory are treatments for the behaviour problems occurring in this condition, because often these are the most problematic area for both people with dementia and their carers.

There has been far too much dependence on drugs to manage these problems in the past. In the future there needs to be much greater emphasis on developing understanding of the problem in the light of the individual's life story and personality.

Development of new medicines

Phase 1
A small number of healthy volunteers, usually between 10 and 12 people, are selected for the first set of trials. These tests work out whether the medicine is safe.

Phase 2
Trials are designed to see if a new medicine works in a small number of patients with the condition or disease being tested. Between 100 and 200 patients are selected and monitored to see if they have mild or severe side effects.

Phase 3
The largest number of patients so far is selected (perhaps between 1,000 and 3,000) to take the medicine under medical supervision for approximately six months. Phase 3 trials are usually carried out in a hospital or clinic setting and may involve a number of different countries.

If the results are satisfactory, they will be presented to the licensing and other relevent authorities who decide whether or not to give them a licence.

Phase 4
Even when newly licensed medicines are launched, they are still tested and many thousands of patients help to continue the research and help doctors. Doctors are looking to see how the new medicine is used in a real-life situation, when a patient is at home or work. If the medicine has a very rare side effect, for example a reaction that will affect one person in 50,000 taking the medicine, then it is extremely unlikely that these side effects will be discovered until after the new medicine is available to be prescribed.

There needs to be more training and research into management of dementia, not involving drugs with their often unpleasant side effects. For example, use of life histories and greater emphasis on looking at behaviours in context may well help reduce reliance on drugs.

KEY POINTS

In the future:

- The numbers of people with dementia will increase

- Greater awareness of the condition and a reduction in stigma may lead to more frequent early diagnosis

- People with dementia should be consulted about decisions involving their care

- Although there is no immediate prospect of a cure, new diagnostic techniques and treatments are being developed

- It will continue to take many years to ensure that a new drug treatment is safe and effective before it becomes widely available

Questions and answers

What is dementia?
Dementia is the general name used to describe the large number of disorders of the brain where there is a progressive deterioration of brain function such as memory, thinking, language and personality.

Is Alzheimer's disease different from dementia?
No. It is not different. Alzheimer's disease *is* a dementia. It is the most common type of dementia. There are many other less common types.

How is a diagnosis of dementia made?
There is no specific test. The diagnosis is usually made either by the GP or by a specialist (psychiatrist or neurologist) who will take a history and ask about the symptoms from both the person with the problem and a close family member/close friend. The history, together with some blood tests, memory tests and possibly a brain scan, will normally make it possible to arrive at a diagnosis.

Can I be tested to see if I have dementia?
A diagnosis is reached in the ways described in answer
to the previous question. If you are worried that you
have dementia, see your doctor to discuss your concerns.

What causes dementia?
The basic cause of all types of dementia is damage to
the nerve cells in the brain. The changes in the brain
depend on the type of dementia, of which the most
common is Alzheimer's disease and the second, but less
common, type is vascular dementia.

In Alzheimer's disease one can see characteristic
abnormalities in the brain called plaques and tangles.
In vascular dementia there is disease of the blood
vessels and evidence of areas of dead tissue in the brain
due to mini-strokes. However, nearly all people with
Alzheimer's disease also have some degree of vascular
disease. Pure vascular dementia is a much less common
type of dementia.

Then there is the question of why some people
develop these diseases and others don't. An individual's
gene structure (inherited factors) may make him or her
more vulnerable to develop Alzheimer's disease, but
there are very few people for whom genes are the only
important cause of this condition.

There must also be a number of environmental and
lifestyle causes of Alzheimer's disease but it has not so
far proved possible to identify conclusively what they are.

How will I know if I am developing dementia?
It has become very common for people to think that
they have a dementia when they forget something.
This is because there is so much greater awareness of

dementia that people talk and worry about it more. You sometimes hear people jokingly saying that they must be getting 'Alzheimer's' when they forget someone's name or telephone number or a film that they have seen recently.

In some cases a person developing dementia is the first to become aware of a memory problem, but usually it is the people around them who are the first to notice. So if you think that you may be susceptible you should be prepared to ask people close to you, or who work with you, if and when they notice a problem with your memory to tell you about it.

Will I get dementia?

We know that the chance of getting dementia increases with age, although we do not know why this is. If there are people in your family who have definitely developed dementia as they have got older, your chance of developing it is slightly greater if you also live to an old age. However, the likelihood that you will die of something completely different is even more likely.

What can I do if I do get dementia?

Don't lose heart. Join the Alzheimer's Society. Find out everything that you can about it. Find other people with dementia to talk to. Don't be afraid to tell people to whom you are close that you have dementia. Try your best to lead as normal a life as possible (for further tips, see 'Living with dementia', page 78)

How can I prevent dementia?

Many people with dementia also have evidence of blood vessel changes. Clots in the blood vessels leading to the heart give rise to heart attacks. Clots in the vessels to the brain can lead to strokes. Large or multiple small strokes can lead to dementia.

Anything that can reduce the formation of blood clots definitely reduces the risk of heart attacks and strokes. So what is good for the heart is good for the brain. We recommend the following:

- A healthy diet – low in saturated fat

- Don't smoke

- Alcohol in moderation

- Regular exercise both physical and mental

- Don't get overweight

- Control diabetes if present

- Control high blood pressure if present

- Keep your mind busy.

There is no guarantee that you will not get dementia if you pay attention to all these factors, but they are good for you anyway!

I have been told that I have dementia. Is there a cure?

No. At this point in time there is no cure. If you are lucky enough to get a good response to drug treatment then it might appear that you are 'cured' for a while. However, these drugs do not affect the disease process so the symptoms will return sooner or later. If they do not it is highly likely that you did not have the correct diagnosis in the first place.

Are there drugs to stop the dementia getting worse?

Yes. There are drugs that help some people with dementia to function better in their everyday lives. They do not help everyone who takes them. We are not yet able to predict who will respond positively.

If a person is helped, the effect of drugs is usually short-lived but this varies from person to person. In people who have responded to drugs it always becomes quite clear at some point that the disease is deteriorating, and when this point arrives there is little point in continuing them.

I have been given a diagnosis of dementia. Can I drive?

Possibly, but you or your family (or sometimes your doctor) will need to notify the Driver and Vehicle Licensing Agency (DVLA) and wait for their decision. The DVLA will ask for a medical report and may decide on the basis of this to renew your licence for a year or revoke your licence. Sometimes they may offer a new driving test to reassess your driving ability.

You would be well advised to start adapting to the idea that you will not be able to carry on driving for too much longer, and start using public transport and taxis or allowing other people to drive you.

Where can I get more information about dementia?

The very best source of information is available from the Alzheimer's Society. GPs or specialists who make a diagnosis of dementia should routinely give you the address, telephone number and website of the Alzheimer's Society. The information is available in printed form and on the internet and there is a helpline available to everyone (see 'Useful information, page 127).

Are there drug trials in which I can take part?

You should ask your GP or specialist if he or she is doing any or if there are any trials being done not too far from where you live. This is also a question that the Alzheimer's Society might be able to help with.

I care for my husband who has dementia. Whom can I ring when I get desperate?

We hope that you will have enough support to make sure that you never get desperate. However, there might well be times when you feel that way. You need to have a list of people whom you can ring by your phone. These should include:

- Your GP

- The named key person in the community mental health team whom you have been seeing

- A friend from your support group with whom you have this arrangement

- Your social worker, if you are getting help from social services

- The helpline of the Alzheimer's Society or Dementia UK

- The chat page on the website of the Alzheimer's Society

- A neighbour or relative with whom you have this arrangement.

My mother is showing worrying signs of memory loss but refuses to go to the doctor and denies that she has a problem. What shall I do?

Try making an appointment yourself with your mother's GP and tell her or him about your concerns. A good GP will listen to you and then probably recommend that you tell your mother that you have been to see the GP and that the GP would like to come and take your mother's blood pressure and do a routine check-up. It is important that you arrange to be present when he or she visits.

My father has dementia. My mother is struggling with everything that she has to do. They adamantly refuse help from outside services. What shall I do?

Do try to persuade your mother to talk with social services. If she won't and there is a problem with money you might be able to help by finding out about and then explaining to them the Attendance Allowance. This is intended to buy extra help so, if your father qualifies, try to persuade your parents to use or allow you to use the money for this purpose. Or you might need to pay for it yourself initially.

You might need to spend time finding someone who can help with the washing, cleaning and shopping. Try to be present the first few times that this person comes to help.

How are we going to choose the right home for my mother who has dementia?

You will want to talk this over with your social worker who might have some homes to suggest to

you. The Alzheimer's Society helpline or the Elderly
Accommodation Council (see 'Useful information',
page 131) might be able to give you a list. However,
lists will only be able to give you names.

If you have access to the internet (you can get this
in a public library), you can look homes up and find
the most recent Care Quality Commission report. If
you do not have access to the internet you can ring
the customer helpline for the Care Quality Commission
(see 'Useful information', page 129) and ask them for
details of recent reports of homes in which you might
be interested. Then you will need to visit some of the
homes that you have chosen and ask some questions.

The Alzheimer's Society has a good factsheet on the
sort of questions that you might want to ask when you
visit a home. You might find it useful to organise for
your mother to spend a day or even a respite admission
in a home that you have found to see how she responds.
This may be a lengthy process but it is well worth
taking time over it.

My mother with dementia needs to go into a home. Who is going to pay for it?
There are three main types of care settings:

1. Extra care sheltered housing

2. Residential homes

3. Nursing homes.

Residential homes do not have to have nurses on
the staff. Nursing homes must employ nurses and be
able to provide 24-hour nursing care. Most homes
are owned by the private sector, some by registered

charities and a very few by the local authorities or the NHS.

Your mother will need to have a multidisciplinary assessment to assess how much care she needs which your local social services department will carry out. This will involve looking at her physical, mental health, social needs and financial resources.

Does not need nursing care

This means that you need to be looking for a residential home. The amount of money that a residential home is going to cost your mother will depend on the local authority's assessment of your mother's financial resources.

If the only money she has is a state pension then the local authority has to make up the difference.

If she has savings over a certain amount (around £23,250 in 2011 but the amount keeps changing) then the savings will be used to help pay for the care. Once savings drop below this amount your mother would be entitled to a financial assessment from social services to determine how much she has to contribute to the cost.

If your mother alone owns a house then the value of the house will be taken into account in the financial assessment.

Needs nursing care

If she is assessed as having nursing needs then she will have a second assessment by the NHS of her registered nursing input needs.

If it is confirmed that she does have nursing needs then the NHS pay the nursing home a flat rate, which at the time of writing is £103.80 per week. This is the amount of money that the NHS will contribute to her care in addition to the money paid by her and the local authority.

In some severe and complex cases the NHS will cover all the costs. This would be applicable if your mother needs constant nursing care and regular supervision by a hospital specialist because she is very frail or severely mentally ill or exhibiting continuous difficult behaviour.

As the carer of my mother with dementia is she or am I entitled to any benefits?

Your mother may be entitled to the Attendance Allowance or the Disability Living Allowance to help with the costs of care. The Attendance Allowance is for people over the age of 65 and the Disability Living Allowance for people under the age of 65. These benefits are not dependent on income or savings and are tax free. As a carer you may also be entitled to a carer's allowance which is paid if you spend more than 35 hours a week caring for someone. However, this may affect other benefits you or your mother receive so check this out.

It is important that you ask advice about this from your social worker, the Alzheimer's Society or your local Citizens Advice Bureau. There is also a freephone Benefits Enquiry Line for people with disabilities, including people with dementia (see 'Useful information', page 126).

You or your mother may be entitled to a reduction in or exemption from the council tax. Ask your council about this.

My father has dementia and is making mistakes with his money. What should I do about this?

If this has not already been done, probably the most important step is for your father (the donor) to make out a lasting power of attorney (LPA), provided that he still has the capacity to do this (see previous chapter, page 84).

This enables a person of his choice (the attorney) to look after his finances when he can no longer do so. It is the responsibility of the attorney to decide when your father is no longer able to manage his financial affairs. If he has any doubts he will ask a doctor for advice.

You can get the necessary forms free from the Office of the Public Guardian (or direct.gov.uk website). These forms are quite complicated and he and you might need help completing them.

You might find it useful to consult a solicitor. The organisation Solicitors for the Elderly specialise in helping people with all kinds of legal advice, including help with the LPA (see page 134). This is expensive but it might be a good deal more expensive not to do this properly. It is important to have a completed LPA made out before the person with dementia no longer has the capacity (mental ability) to do this.

If you want to set up a power of attorney an independent person needs to sign a declaration that you understand and agree to this. This may be a person whom you have known for over two years or a professional such as a doctor.

If this person has any doubt about your father's capacity, you should ask his doctor or local old age psychiatrist to make a capacity assessment. Capacity in this case means that your father is able to understand what the LPA involves and can choose a person whom he trusts to look after his finances.

There are a number of other practical things that you can do if he agrees, such as making arrangements with his bank to allow him to withdraw only small amounts of money at a time, organising for bills and pensions to be paid direct from the bank, telling the local shops of his problem. In this way you can help your father to remain independent for as long as possible without making expensive mistakes.

I'm worried that my mother's neighbour is regularly taking money from her. My mum is very confused now. What can I do?

In addition to protecting your mother's money as outlined in the question above, this may be a case of financial exploitation. Your local social services have a duty to investigate this using a procedure called safeguarding. You can raise an alert by speaking to your mother's social worker or the local social services duty team.

The doctor has told me that my wife has Alzheimer's disease. He told me that he had explained to her what the problem was but had not used the diagnostic label. What shall I tell her?

In our experience it is always helpful to tell the person that he or she has a form of dementia called Alzheimer's disease. You might want to do this yourself or ask your doctor to do it.

If you do this yourself you need to go on to say that this will not progress rapidly but as time goes on she will need more help with everyday activities, and you and others will be there to help and support her.

The distress that you feel you might be causing is often lessened by the fact that your wife might well forget what she has been told. Furthermore, some people are even quite relieved to have a name to give their problem, which is otherwise puzzling.

How your brain works

The conscious and subconscious

The brain is by far the most complex and sophisticated organ in the body. It enables us to think, remember, move around, speak, interpret vision, sound, smell, taste and touch, and make decisions. These processes are all conscious; in other words we are aware of these events.

The brain also performs a lot of subconscious tasks of which we are not aware. For example, it controls our vital body systems such as breathing, heart and blood pressure. It also produces various hormones that regulate our metabolism and other body systems.

Anatomy of the brain

The healthy adult brain weighs about 1.3 kilograms (about 2 pounds) and is thought to contain about 100 billion nerve cells called neurons. Once we reach adolescence, the brain does not create any new neurons.

The central nervous system

The brain and spinal cord form the central nervous system (CNS). The brain performs many complex functions, for instance it is the source of our consciousness, intelligence and creativity. It also monitors and controls, through the peripheral nervous system (PNS), most body processes – ranging from the automatic, such as breathing, to complex voluntary activities, such as riding a bicycle.

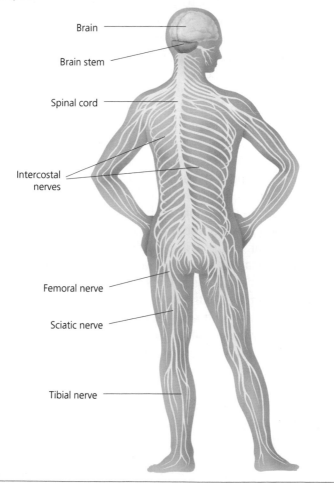

Brain

Brain stem

Spinal cord

Intercostal nerves

Femoral nerve

Sciatic nerve

Tibial nerve

The size and structure of these neurons vary depending on the role that they play. For example, neurons responsible for movement are very different to those that interpret vision.

Neurons allow messages to be transmitted between different parts of the brain and to the rest of the body by tiny electrical impulses. Rather than just a big mass of neurons, the brain is highly organised into different areas, which communicate with each other via bundles of neurons called tracts. The result is a web of highly organised connections.

Nerve transmission

Neurons connect to each other through tiny spaces between nerve cells called synapses. Neurons have between 1,000 and 10,000 synapses and are constantly communicating with each other by releasing chemicals called neurotransmitters. (You are able to understand what you are reading in this book because nerve cells are firing messages and releasing neurotransmitters.)

When an electrical impulse travels down a neuron, synapses will be activated to release a small amount of neurotransmitter. There are many different neurotransmitters with different functions. For example, some neurotransmitters activate the next nerve cell in the chain, whereas others inhibit it.

Whatever their function, all neurons have a similar structure. The centre of the neuron is the nucleus. Typically, several short fibres called dendrites run to the nucleus. These transmit nerve impulses to the centre. A single fibre, called an axon, transmits nerve impulses away from the nucleus.

How nerve cells transmit signals

Essentially, your brain is like a bundle of telephone wires transmitting and receiving messages within your brain and to and from other parts of your body. Some of the messages are sent by electrical impulses; others depend on the release and transmission of particular chemicals called neurotransmitters.

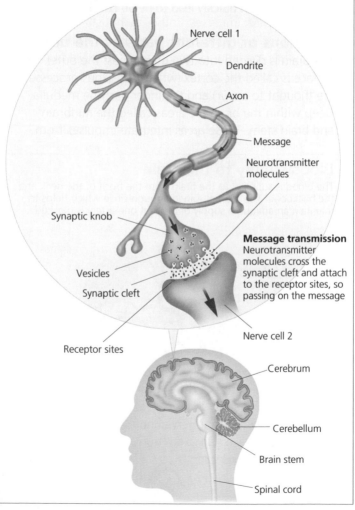

Nerve cell 1

Dendrite

Axon

Message

Neurotransmitter molecules

Synaptic knob

Message transmission
Neurotransmitter molecules cross the synaptic cleft and attach to the receptor sites, so passing on the message

Vesicles

Synaptic cleft

Nerve cell 2

Receptor sites

Cerebrum

Cerebellum

Brain stem

Spinal cord

To stay healthy, the brain requires a lot of oxygen and glucose, which is supplied by large blood vessels (the carotid and vertebral arteries). About a litre of blood (about one-fifth of the heart's output) passes through the brain every minute. Any interruption to the blood supply can quickly lead to nerve cell damage.

Functions of different parts of the brain

The brain is divided into two main areas: the outer surface is called the cortex (where conscious processes are thought to occur) and the inner part the medulla. Deep within the brain are areas called the midbrain and brain stem. These areas integrate impulses from

Blood supply to the brain

The blood is supplied to the brain from the front of the neck and the backbone. The arteries join in a rough circle which helps to maintain an adequate supply of blood if one artery is blocked.

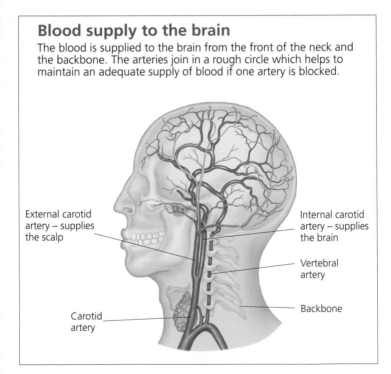

External carotid artery – supplies the scalp

Internal carotid artery – supplies the brain

Vertebral artery

Backbone

Carotid artery

different parts of the brain and information coming from the rest of the body (rather like a complex telephone exchange) and control our subconscious processes such as blood pressure and heart rate. The cerebellum, located near the back of the brain, helps control movement.

The cortex

The cortex, on the surface of the brain, is divided into different areas, called lobes, which have different

The human brain

The brain is encased in the bony skull and communicates with the rest of the body through the cranial nerves (which pass through openings in the skull) and the spinal nerves (whch pass from the spinal cord through small gaps between the bones of the spine) and control the arms, trunk and legs.

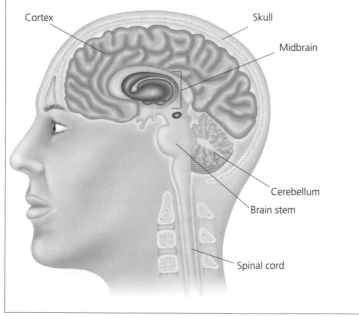

Cortex

Skull

Midbrain

Cerebellum

Brain stem

Spinal cord

functions. Although it is probably over-simplifying the brain function somewhat, it is useful to know what lobes are important in different processes in the brain.

Frontal lobes

The frontal lobe (the largest lobe, sitting over the front half of the brain) has many functions including abstract thinking, planning and making decisions. It is thought to be the area that controls urges and behaviours; some people who have damage to the frontal lobes may become disinhibited and do strange or embarrassing things; others may become unmotivated and apathetic. The back part of the frontal lobe is where voluntary movement is controlled.

Parietal lobe

Behind the frontal lobe is the parietal lobe. This is involved in interpreting touch and hearing, and collects information from other sensory systems (such as vision) to help us integrate different sensations. Damage to the parietal lobe can result in someone not being able to understand sensory inputs.

Temporal lobe

The temporal lobe is tucked underneath the frontal and parietal lobes and is thought to be the main site for memory, but is also involved in hearing and understanding speech. People with damage to the temporal lobe may have great difficulty in remembering things. A part of the temporal lobe called the hippocampus, sometimes regarded as the main seat of memory, is affected early in Alzheimer's disease.

The structure of the brain

The brain has two hemispheres: the left and the right. Each hemisphere is composed of four lobes. Each of the four lobes of each cerebral hemisphere has its own particular physical and mental functions. These can be impaired by brain damage.

SIDE VIEW

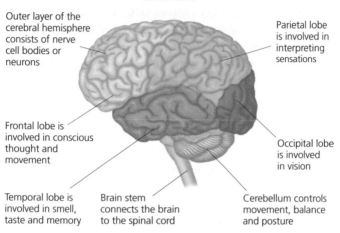

Outer layer of the cerebral hemisphere consists of nerve cell bodies or neurons

Parietal lobe is involved in interpreting sensations

Frontal lobe is involved in conscious thought and movement

Occipital lobe is involved in vision

Temporal lobe is involved in smell, taste and memory

Brain stem connects the brain to the spinal cord

Cerebellum controls movement, balance and posture

TOP VIEW

Right hemisphere

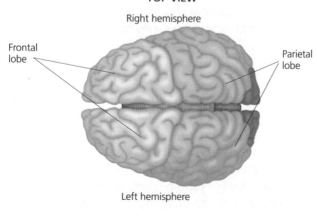

Frontal lobe

Parietal lobe

Left hemisphere

Occipital lobe

At the back of the brain is the occipital lobe, which is the main part of the brain involved in interpretation of vision.

Memory

Memory is the process of registering new information, storing it and recalling it when needed. We are constantly laying down new memories.

Scientists have suggested there are two main types of memory.

Short-term memory

'Short-term memory' retains a small amount of information (about seven items) for up to 30 seconds. For example, we can often remember a new phone number or car registration number for just long enough to write it down, but if something else happens we quickly forget this information.

Long-term memory

Memories can move from short-term to 'long-term' memory. Memories may move into the long-term memory because we repeat the fact again and again (such as learning lines for a play) or the memory is associated with a strong emotion. For instance, most people can recall incidents that made them very upset or frightened. This is known as 'flashbulb' memory.

Memory can also be classified according to the type of information stored. Procedural memory requires no conscious effort to recall. It often refers to routine things that we do. For example, an experienced car driver would not have to think 'how do I use this?' when he or she gets behind the wheel.

Declarative (or explicit) memory does require conscious effort – if you want to drive to see a friend you need to consciously remember what his or her address is. Declarative memory is sometimes further divided into semantic and episodic memory.

Semantic memory encodes general facts, not related to a particular time or place or context. Episodic memory is related to a particular context. For example, remembering that someone is your friend would be semantic memory, but recalling that you last saw him or her when you visited the seaside on a hot Saturday afternoon last summer would be episodic memory.

Effect of dementias on brain structure and function

One of the hallmarks of most kinds of dementia is shrinkage of the brain. This is thought to be due to the dying off of some of the nerve cells. In most kinds of dementia, the amount of some chemicals in the brain is reduced, leading to problems with nerve cells communicating with each other.

The loss of nerve cells combined with loss of chemicals results in symptoms such as loss of memory, change in personality, and difficulties in thinking, planning and language.

Although it may vary from person to person, most people with dementia will develop problems with memory first. The ability to store new memories declines, often subtly at first. Frequently, more recent memories are often lost first in dementia. Memories from childhood may remain well after someone has forgotten recent events.

Brain of someone with Alzheimer's disease

Computer graphic of a vertical (coronal) slice through the brain of an Alzheimer's disease patient (left) compared with a normal brain (right). The Alzheimer's disease brain is considerably shrunken, due to the degeneration and death of nerve cells. Apart from a decrease in brain volume, the surface of the brain is often more deeply folded. Tangled protein filaments (neurofibrillary tangles) occur within nerve cells and patients also develop brain lesions of beta-amyloid protein.

Alzheimer's disease brain   Healthy brain

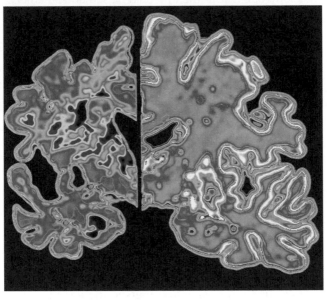

KEY POINTS

■ The brain is a complex organ with a highly organised network of 100 billion nerve cells

■ Brain cells communicate with each other using chemicals called neurotransmitters

■ In dementia there is a reduction of nerve cells and neurotransmitters

Useful information

Useful addresses

We have included the following organisations because, on preliminary investigation, they may be of use to the reader. However, we do not have first-hand experience of each organisation and so cannot guarantee the organisation's integrity. The reader must therefore exercise his or her own discretion and judgement when making further enquiries.

Age UK

York House, 207–221 Pentonville Road
London N1 9UZ
Tel: 020 7239 1983
Age UK Advice: 0800 169 6565
Website: www.ageuk.org.uk

Can provide practical help. Researches into the needs of older people and is involved in policy-making. Provides advice on a range of subjects for people aged over 50. Publishes books and offers services via local branches

Alzheimer's Disease International
64 Great Suffolk Street, London SE1 0BL
Tel: 020 7981 0880
Website: www.alz.co.uk

Umbrella organisation for Alzheimer's disease
associations around the world.

Alzheimer Society of Ireland
Temple Road, Blackrock, Co. Dublin, Ireland
Tel: +353 (0)1 207 3800
Helpline: 1800 341 341
Website: www.alzheimer.ie

Aims to maximise quality of life by providing services
and information for people affected by Alzheimer's
disease and other dementias.

Alzheimer Scotland – Action on Dementia
22 Drumsheugh Gardens, Edinburgh EH3 7RN
Tel: 0131 243 1453
Helpline: 0808 808 3000
Website: www.alzscot.org.uk

Provides advice, support and local services in Scotland
for people with dementia and their carers.

Alzheimer's Society
Devon House, 58 St Katharine's Way, London E1W 1JX
Tel: 020 7423 3500
Helpline: 0845 300 0336
Website: www.alzheimers.org.uk

Care and research charity supplying information and

support for people with dementia and their carers.
There are branches in Northern Ireland and Wales.

Benefits Enquiry Line

Tel: 0800 882200
Minicom: 0800 243355
Website: www.dwp.gov.uk
N. Ireland: 0800 220674

Government agency giving information and advice
on sickness and disability benefits for people with
disabilities and their carers.

Carers UK

20 Great Dover Street, London SE1 4LX
Tel: 020 7378 4999
Helpline: 0808 808 7777 (Wed, Thurs 10am–12 noon,
2–4pm)
Website: www.carersuk.org

Encourages carers to recognise their own needs. Offers
information, advice and support to all people who are
unpaid carers looking after others with medical or other
problems. Branches organise activities to help carers,
social events and helplines.

Citizens Advice Bureaux

Myddelton House, 115–123 Pentonville Road
London N1 9LZ
Tel: 020 7833 2181 (admin only)
Website: www.adviceguide.org.uk

HQ of national charity offering a wide variety of
practical, financial and legal advice. Network of local

charities throughout the UK listed in phone books and in *Yellow Pages* under 'Counselling and Advice'.

CJD Support Network
PO Box 346, Market Drayton, Shropshire TF9 4WN
Tel: 01630 673993
Helpline: 01630 673973
Website: www.cjdsupport.net

Provides help and support for people with all strains of Creutzfeldt–Jakob disease (CJD), their carers and concerned professionals. Runs a national helpline and can help families in financial need.

Clinical Knowledge Summaries
Sowerby Centre for Health Informatics at Newcastle (SCHIN Ltd), Clayton House, Clayton Road, Jesmond Newcastle upon Tyne NE2 1TL
Tel: 0845 113 1000
Website: www.schin.co.uk

A website mainly for GPs giving information for patients listed by disease plus named self-help organisations.

Care Quality Commission
National Correspondence, Citygate, Gallowgate
Newcastle upon Tyne NE1 4PA
Tel: 0300 061 6161 (Mon–Fri 8.30am–5.30pm)
Website: www.cqc.org.uk

The official body regulating care homes and agencies that provide nurses or care workers who carry out personal tasks.

Counsel and Care

Twyman House, 16 Bonny Street, London NW1 9PG
Tel: 020 7241 8555 (Mon–Fri 9am–5pm)
Helpline: 0845 300 7585
Website: www.counselandcare.org.uk

Voice for all older people and their families. Advises on a number of issues, including community care, welfare benefits and hospital discharge.

Court of Protection

See Office of the Public Guardian.

Crossroads Care

Attendants Schemes, 10 Regent Place, Rugby, Warwickshire CV21 2PN
Tel: 0845 450 0350
Website: www.crossroads.org.uk

Aims to improve the lives of carers by giving practical support and providing a paid, trained person to offer respite care in the home.

Dementia UK

6 Camden High Street, London NW1 0JH
Tel: 020 7874 7200
Helpline: 0845 257 9406
Website: www.dementiauk.org.uk

Focuses on providing specialist dementia nurses who can offer practical advice, emotional support and skills to families and carers of people with dementia.

DVLA (Driver and Vehicle Licensing Agency)
Swansea SA6 7JL
Helpline: 0300 790 6806
Website: www.dvla.gov.uk

Government office providing advice for drivers with special needs.

Elderly Accommodation Council
3rd Floor, 89 Albert Embankment, London SE1 7TP
Advice line: 0800 377 7070
Website: www.housingcare.org

A source of information on all forms of accommodation for older people.

Huntington's Disease Association
Neurosupport Centre, Norton Street
Liverpool L3 8LR
Tel: 0151 298 3298
Website: www.hda.org.uk

Offers support and understanding to anyone affected by Huntington's disease. Has a network of regional care advisers who provide information, workshops and educational services.

National Council for Palliative Care
The Fitzpatrick Building, 188–194 York Way, London N7 9AS
Tel: 020 7697 1520
Website: www.ncpc.org.uk

Promotes the extension and improvement of palliative care services for all people with life-threatening and life-limiting conditions.

National Institute for Health and Clinical Excellence (NICE)
MidCity Place, 71 High Holborn
London WC1V 6NA
Tel: 020 7067 5800
Website: www.nice.org.uk

Provides national guidance on the promotion of good health and the prevention and treatment of ill-health. Patient information leaflets are available for each piece of guidance issued.

Office of the Public Guardian
PO Box 15118
Birmingham B16 6QX
Tel: 0300 456 0300
Website: www.direct.gov.uk

Responsible for providing services that promote the financial and social well-being of people with mental incapacity.

Parkinson's UK
National Office, 215 Vauxhall Bridge Road
London SW1V 1EJ
Tel: 020 7931 8080
Helpline: 0808 800 0303
Website: www.parkinsons.org.uk

Provides information and support for people with Parkinson's disease and their carers. Offers advice on living with Parkinson's disease, and the drug, surgery and therapy options available.

Princess Royal Trust for Carers
Unit 14, Bourne Court, Southend Road, Woodford Green, Essex IG8 8HD
Tel: 0844 800 4361
Website: www.carers.org and www.youngcarers.net

Largest provider of comprehensive support services for carers in the UK. Provides quality information, advice and support services to carers, including young carers. Also has offices in Scotland, Wales and northern England.

Useful links
BBC
www.bbc.co.uk/health
A helpful website: easy to navigate and offers lots of useful advice and information. Also contains links to other related topics.

Healthtalkonline
www.healthtalkonline.org
A website for carers which includes interviews of carers of people with dementia.

Lewy Body Society
www.lewybody.org
Raises awareness and educates the public, the medical profession and those in health-care decision-making positions about dementia with Lewy bodies.

Patient UK
www.patient.co.uk
Patient care website.

Pick's Disease Support Group
www.pdsg.org.uk
Information and support for carers of people with Pick's disease. The website doesn't give a contact address but does give contact details for committee members in different areas of the UK.

Solicitors for the Elderly (SFE)
www.solicitorsfortheelderly.com
A national organisation of lawyers, such as solicitors, barristers and legal executives, who are committed to providing and promoting robust, comprehensive and independent legal advice for older people, their family and carers.

Further reading
The Alzheimer's Society produces *Living with Dementia* – a monthly magazine – and a wide range of practical information and advice sheets and a list of publications about all aspects of dementia and living with dementia. Many of these are available on the Society's website: www.alzheimers.org.uk

The 36 Hour Day: A family guide to caring for people with Alzheimer's disease, other dementias, and memory loss in later life, 4th edn, by Nancy L. Mace. Baltimore, MA: Johns Hopkins University Press, 2006.

Alzheimer's and Other Dementias: Answers at your fingertips, 3rd edn, by Harry Cayton, Nori Graham, James Warner. London: Class Health Publishing, 2008.

Dancing with Dementia: *My story of living positively with dementia*, by Christine Bryden. London: Jessica Kingsley Publishers, 2005.

The internet as a further source of information

After reading this book, you may feel that you would like further information on the subject. The internet is of course an excellent place to look and there are many websites with useful information about medical disorders, related charities and support groups.

For those who do not have a computer at home some bars and cafes offer facilities for accessing the internet. These are listed in the Yellow Pages under 'Internet Bars and Cafes' and 'Internet Providers'. Your local library offers a similar facility and has staff to help you find the information that you need.

It should always be remembered, however, that the internet is unregulated and anyone is free to set up a website and add information to it. Many websites offer impartial advice and information that has been compiled and checked by qualified medical professionals. Some, on the other hand, are run by commercial organisations with the purpose of promoting their own products. Others still are run by pressure groups, some of which will provide carefully assessed and accurate information whereas others may be suggesting medications or treatments that are not supported by the medical and scientific community.

Unless you know the address of the website you want to visit – for example, www.familydoctor.co.uk – you may find the following guidelines useful when searching the internet for information.

Search engines and other searchable sites

Google (www.google.co.uk) is the most popular search engine used in the UK, followed by Yahoo! (http://uk.yahoo.com) and MSN (www.msn.co.uk). Also popular are the search engine provided by Internet Service Providers such as TalkTalk and other sites such as the BBC site (www.bbc.co.uk).

In addition to the search engines that index the whole web, there are also medical sites with search facilities, which act almost like mini-search engines, but cover only medical topics or even a particular area of medicine. Again, it is wise to look at who is responsible for compiling the information offered to ensure that it is impartial and medically accurate. The NHS Direct site (www.nhsdirect.nhs.uk) is an example of a searchable medical site.

Links to many British medical charities can be found at the Association of Medical Research Charities website (www.amrc.org.uk) and at Charity Choice (www.charitychoice.co.uk).

Search phrases

Be specific when entering a search phrase. Searching for information on 'cancer' will return results for many different types of cancer as well as on cancer in general. You may even find sites offering astrological information. More useful results will be returned by using search phrases such as 'lung cancer' and 'treatments for lung cancer'. Both Google and Yahoo! offer an advanced search option that includes the ability to search for the exact phrase, enclosing the search phrase in quotes, that is, 'treatments for lung cancer' will have the same effect. Limiting a search to an exact phrase reduces the number of results returned but it is best to refine a search to an exact match only if you are not getting useful results with a normal search. Adding 'UK' to your search term will bring up mainly British sites, so a good phrase might be 'lung cancer' UK (don't include UK within the quotes).

Always remember the internet is international and unregulated. It holds a wealth of valuable information but individual sites may be biased, out of date or just plain wrong. Family Doctor Publications accepts no responsibility for the content of links published in this series.

Index

Your pages

We have included the following pages because they may help you manage your illness or condition and its treatment.

Before an appointment with a health professional, it can be useful to write down a short list of questions of things that you do not understand, so that you can make sure that you do not forget anything.

Some of the sections may not be relevant to your circumstances.

We are always pleased to receive constructive criticism or suggestions about how to improve the books. You can contact us at:

Email: familydoctor@btinternet.com
Letter: Family Doctor Publications
          PO Box 4664
          Poole
          BH15 1NN

Thank you

Health-care contact details

Name:

Job title:

Place of work:

Tel:

Name:

Job title:

Place of work:

Tel:

Name:

Job title:

Place of work:

Tel:

Name:

Job title:

Place of work:

Tel:

Significant past health events – illnesses/operations/investigations/treatments

Event	Month	Year	Age (at time)

Appointments for health care

Name:

Place:

Date:

Time:

Tel:

Name:

Place:

Date:

Time:

Tel:

Name:

Place:

Date:

Time:

Tel:

Name:

Place:

Date:

Time:

Tel:

Appointments for health care

Name:

Place:

Date:

Time:

Tel:

Name:

Place:

Date:

Time:

Tel:

Name:

Place:

Date:

Time:

Tel:

Name:

Place:

Date:

Time:

Tel:

Current medication(s) prescribed by your doctor

Medicine name:

Purpose:

Frequency & dose:

Start date:

End date:

Medicine name:

Purpose:

Frequency & dose:

Start date:

End date:

Medicine name:

Purpose:

Frequency & dose:

Start date:

End date:

Medicine name:

Purpose:

Frequency & dose:

Start date:

End date:

Other medicines/supplements you are taking, not prescribed by your doctor

Medicine/treatment:

Purpose:

Frequency & dose:

Start date:

End date:

Medicine/treatment:

Purpose:

Frequency & dose:

Start date:

End date:

Medicine/treatment:

Purpose:

Frequency & dose:

Start date:

End date:

Medicine/treatment:

Purpose:

Frequency & dose:

Start date:

End date:

Questions to ask at appointments
(Note: do bear in mind that doctors work under great time pressure, so long lists may not be helpful for either of you)